Private Practice in
Audiology and Speech Pathology

Private Practice in Audiology and Speech Pathology

Edited by

R. Ray Battin, Ph.D.
Director, Battin Clinic, Houston, Texas

Donna R. Fox, Ph.D.
Professor, School of Communication,
University of Houston, Houston, Texas

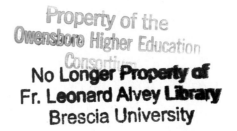
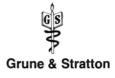

Grune & Stratton

A Subsidiary of Harcourt Brace Jovanovich, Publishers

New York   San Francisco   London

Library of Congress Cataloging in Publication Data
Main entry under title:

Private practice in audiology and speech pathology.

   Bibliography: p.
   Includes index.
    1.   Speech, Disorders of—Practice.   2.   Audiology
—Practice.   I.   Battin, R. Ray.   II.   Fox, Donna
Russell.
RC423.P78   616.8′55   78-12494
ISBN 0-8089-1132-5

Grune & Stratton, Inc.
111 Fifth Avenue
New York, New York 10003

Distributed in the United Kingdom by
Academic Press, Inc. (London) Ltd.
24/28 Oval Road, London NW1

Library of Congress Catalog Number 78-12494

International Standard Book Number 0-8089-1132-5

Printed in the United States of America

Contents

ACKNOWLEDGMENTS   vi
PREFACE   vii
CONTRIBUTORS   viii

INTRODUCTION   1

PART I

  I.   Opening the Doors   9
      R. Ray Battin and Donna R. Fox

 II. Business Aspects of the Practice   27
      R. Ray Battin and John L. Boland

III. A Consideration of Outpatient Speech and Language
      Pathology Services Under Medicare   53
      H. Aubrey Feiwell

 IV. Forensic Speech Pathology   73
      Donna R. Fox

PART II

  V. The Clinical Aspects of Speech and Language Pathology   91
      Donna R. Fox and R. Ray Battin

 VI. Report Writing for Private Practitioners   115
      Kenneth J. Knepflar

VII. Speech Pathology Services in Home Care Agencies   137
      Nona Lee Barr

PART III

VIII. Clinical Aspects of Audiology   191
      Roy C. Rowland, Jr.

 IX. Electronystagmography: Its Role and Function in Audiological
      Private Practice   241
      Darrell L. Teter

  X. Dispensing Hearing Aids in Private Practice   283
      Vernon C. Bragg

Index   305

Acknowledgments

We wish to express our sincere appreciation to Susan Freitag for her excellent editorial and literary assistance and to Marianne Hagg from the Office of Research Administration of the University of Houston for her care in the preparation of this manuscript.

We are especially grateful to the contributors who took time from their busy practices to share their expertise and experiences.

R. Ray Battin, Ph.D.
Donna R. Fox, Ph.D.

Preface

One must develop a philosophy of self as a professional person, as a clinician dealing with behavior change. This is unlike the philosophy of a teacher in that the work clinicians do is best described as habilitation. This does not mean that the clinician does not need to have a thorough understanding of learning, however, since clinicians must understand learning theory as it applies to the clinical setting. Too often, clinicians are described as tutors or speech teachers. If the title "speech language pathologist" or "audiologist" is not encompassing enough, that of "specialist dealing with speech, language, and hearing disorders" more aptly covers the field than do teacher, correctionist, or therapist.

We intend this book to be used by speech pathologists or audiologists in private practice. While it may also be helpful to the clinician in other environments, we have geared the contents primarily to the special needs of the private practitioner and stressed the clinical aspect of the profession.

Contributors

Nona Lee Barr, M.A.
Director of Speech Pathology
Home Health Services of Louisiana, Inc.
New Orleans, Louisiana
Private Practice
Metairie, Louisiana

R. Ray Battin, Ph.D.
Director of The Battin Clinic
Houston, Texas
Clinical Instructor
University of Texas Medical School
Galveston, Texas

John L. Boland, Ph.D.
Director of the Oklahoma Psychological and Educational Center
Oklahoma City, Oklahoma
Instructor, Rehabilitation Medicine
University of Oklahoma Medical School
Oklahoma City, Oklahoma

Vernon C. Bragg, Ph.D.
Clinical Audiologist in private practice
San Antonio, Texas

H. Aubrey Feiwell, M.A.
Speech Pathologist in private practice
Bloomfield Hills, Michigan
President, H. Aubrey Feiwell, P.C.
Bloomfield Hills, Michigan

Kenneth J. Knepflar, Ph.D.
Speech Pathologist in private practice
Pasadena, California

Donna R. Fox, Ph.D.
Professor, School of Communication
University of Houston
Private Practice
Kelsey Seybold Clinic
Houston, Texas

Roy C. Rowland, Jr., Ph.D.
Private practice in audiology
Oklahoma City, Oklahoma

Darrell L. Teter, Ph.D.
Private practice in audiology and speech pathology
Denver, Colorado

INTRODUCTION

R. Ray Battin, Ph.D. and Donna R. Fox, Ph.D

Private or independent practice in the area of speech pathology and audiology has existed as long as the profession itself. Renowned practitioners such as Bleumel, Froeschels, Brodnitz, Weis, and others have not only maintained an independent practice, but have also contributed to the literature and have been active in training in their areas of specialization. Many or most of these men held medical degrees, and we must remember that it is in the area of medicine that clinical skills are acknowledged. Those moving through the academic degree program have tended to minimize this aspect of our profession and instead become researchers and academicians, leaving the clinical work to lesser trained individuals. As a result, our medical colleagues have received acclaim in our specialty while we have been lax in displaying and rewarding clinical skill.

Paul Knight has practiced speech pathology independently in the Chicago area for more than 30 years. He is probably the most experienced and best known private practitioner, and has been active in the state speech and hearing association as well as the American Speech and Hearing Association (ASHA). He was one of the founding members of the American Academy of Private Practice in Speech Pathology and Audiology. In 1947, he published an article on private practice, which was later published as a chapter in Speech Therapy: A Book of Readings, edited by Charles Van Riper. In 1959, Raymond Summers reported that 32% of public school therapists in Indiana engaged in some private practice. Landis and Battin surveyed speech

and hearing personnel in Texas in 1962, and
found a 40.8% participation in private practice. At that time they concluded, "Clearly,
a private practice is fast contributing to
the growing pains of the young profession of
speech therapy/correction/pathology. It must
be studied, understood in proper perspective,
and ultimately regulated before the practice
of speech (pathology) can observe and enjoy a
professional stature comparable to that of
related professions."

To this end, ASHA appointed an ad hoc
committee on private practice. Paul Knight
was the first chairman, and during his tenure
the committee undertook to do a comprehensive
study of private practice. This was reported
in 1961 in the ASHA Journal. Following this,
the committee presented its recommendations
for basic requirements in training and experience for the individual entering private
practice.

Since that article was published the
image of the private practitioner has emerged
with greater clarity. In 1964, an official
ASHA survey indicated that 2% of individuals
in our profession engaged substantially (30
or more hours a week) in private practice.
While no further official survey results have
appeared, a number of factors have combined
to increase the interest in the work setting
of the private practitioner. Two major
factors are: (1) the additional numbers of
speech pathologists and audiologists available for the work market, and (2) the advent
of national legislation regarding the delivery of health care services, including many
of the helping professions such as speech
pathology and audiology.

The year 1965 saw the birth of the
Academy of Private Practice, which was organized as, and originally called, Speech

Pathologists and Audiologists in Private Practice. Its name was changed to the American Academy of Private Practice in Speech Pathology and Audiology when it was incorporated as a nonprofit organization. This organization grew from the need of individuals in private practice to have a means of ongoing education in clinical methods as well as discussion of the business and management aspects of operating an independent practice. The California Speech Pathologists/Audiologists in Private Practice (CALSPAPP) was an offshoot of the original Speech Pathologists and Audiologists in Private Practice (SPAPP) organization. This has been an active state organization that has provided strong programs not only for the independent practitioner, but for anyone in the clinical areas of speech pathology and audiology.

The Academy set forth the following as minimum requirements for the individual entering independent practice:

1. Holds the earned doctorate degree, based in part on a program of studies primarily in the field of speech pathology and/or audiology. The degree must have been awarded by an accredited university offering specialization in these fields.

2. Has acquired, since the beginning of graduate study, not less than five years of paid full-time or equivalent part-time professional clinical experience in rendering speech pathology and/or audiology services. Two of these years must have been acquired subsequent to receiving the doctorate degree. Also during this time, he has had major responsibility for the clinical management of patients of all ages with a wide range in degree and variety of disorders in his area of competence.

3. Holds the Certificate of Clinical Competence, in the area in which he practices, awarded by the American Speech and Hearing Association.

To the individual with a newly acquired masters degree, the above standards may appear excessive. However, the private practice setting is not the place to acquire clinical skills. D'Asaro (1971) stated that the unique features of private practice consist mainly of "the fee relationship, the regular family contacts, and the potential intensification of the therapeutic relationship afforded by the private practice." These factors require the expertise of the seasoned clinician. A mature individual who has developed a personal ethic and can handle the transference of affection which develops on the part of the clinician as well as the patient, and who understands the roles the parent, patient, and clinician must play as they interact with each other will make fewer errors in the therapeutic setting.

This unique setting for the delivery of speech and hearing services has emphasized the need for a re-evaluation of the concept of ethics. Webster defines ethics as "the discipline dealing with what is good and bad and with moral duty and obligation; a set of principles or values." Our national organization subscribes to a code of ethics that may be in need of expansion so that more specific guidelines will be available to the individual practioner.

REFERENCES

D'Asaro MJ: Who is private practice? The California Journal of Communication Disorders I:17-24, 1971

Knight PD: Advantages and disadvantages of private practice. Journal of Speech Disorders 12:199-201, 1947

Knight PD, et al.: Private practice in speech pathology and audiology. Asha 3(2): 387-406, 1961

Landis BA, Battin RR: Private practice in speech therapy in Texas. Southern Speech Journal 27:284-289, 1962

Summers R: Private practice of public school therapists in Indiana. Journal of Speech and Hearing Disorders 24:41-54, 1959

Van Riper C, ed: Speech Therapy: A Book of Readings. New York, Prentice-Hall, 1953, pp. 287-290

PART I

CHAPTER I

OPENING THE DOORS

R. Ray Battin, Ph.D. and Donna R. Fox, Ph.D.

To be in private practice, a speech pathologist or audiologist must be both rigid and flexible. He must be rigid in demanding that only the best possible care is given to his patients. A part of this will come through his restricting his activities to areas where he is well-trained, interested, and skilled, and this also applies to any staff members that he may have in his clinic. It is imperative that he monitor their performance so that they, too, are working only in the areas in which they are trained, skilled, and interested. He must be flexible in allowing himself to grow professionally, taking on educational work with professional colleagues, and referring quickly and willingly those patients who do not fit into his treatment or clinical program. Too often, in the beginning of a practice, the individual finds himself a generalist, and patients on the fringes of his capabilities receive poor or inadequate care. As one becomes more comfortable in practice, more specialization emerges. It is a shame that we do not have more specialization at the beginning, with expansion as one acquires clinical skills and broadens one's horizons.

The means of initiating a private practice rest with the individual. A first prerequisite, no matter what the means, is adequate capital to provide for living expenses for at least three years. Some estimate three to five years before a return is realized on one's investment. This does not

mean that no money is coming in during this
period of time, but rather that it takes this
long to build a practice, pay out the initial
outlay, maintain ongoing expenses, and realize a stable income. The individual contem-
plating private practice should examine all
of the alternatives. These range from solo
practice, in which one literally hangs out a
shingle and waits for patients, to entering
an established group practice or setting up a
new group practice with others.

Beginning Practice

When the practitioner decides that
private practice is the environment in which
he wishes to deliver service, several variables must be defined in order to initiate
the practice. These are: (1) work time, (2)
form, (3) setting, and (4) types of patients.

With regard to work time, part-time
practice often provides a means of beginning
to practice privately. Generally, the practitioner is employed by a group or an institution, and then sees private patients outside of this primary work setting. In such a
case, the clinician delivering the service is
actually in part-time private practice, as is
the consultant who contracts time to see
patients for clinics, hospitals, and school
systems. If the delivery of such services is
the responsibility of an individual, no
matter how large or how small the time involved, such an individual is within the
realm of the private practice concept.

In the ASHA survey of 1964, 24% of the
87% who responded to the survey questionnaire
engaged in some degree of private practice.
By now this number has probably increased;
that is, if we accept the concept of private
practice as a fee-for-service relationship

between the clinician and the patient. Frequently, a practitioner will begin on a part-time basis and increase his private practice until this form of service delivery has become a full-time position.

The second variable in private practice is the form in which the individual may practice. There are a number of legal defin- itions and many personal preferences. These vary from the individual practitioner who chooses to do only consultative work, to the individual who practices in an office within a large complex, to the individual who moves from setting to setting.

The form of the practice may be totally individual (a one-person practice) or a complex liaison among members of a group. In the individual practice, the form may be built upon the special talents and responsi- bility of a single person. He may move from office to office or hospital to hospital, or he may maintain only an answering service or a post office box number. An alternative form is the proprietorship, in which one individual owns the practice and retains control of the services, but employs others, often in other disciplines. Another form of practice is the partnership, in which two or more individuals combine their talents. This is a legal arrangement and the two henceforth are responsible, both ethically and finan- cially. Still another form is the corpora- tion, in which three or more individuals combine under the legal definition of a corporation.

The third variable to be considered in setting up a private practice is that of setting. The setting may vary; it may be a post office box for clinicians who see their patients in places other than an office, an individual office paid for by the individual

practitioner, or shared facilities in which
an office may be used on alternate days by,
for example, a psychiatrist, a psychologist,
or another professional, together with the
speech pathologist or audiologist. This may
involve more than one location if an individual's practice extends throughout a large
metropolitan area. For example, on Mondays
and Wednesdays, the speech pathologist may
use one office while a psychiatrist uses an
office in another part of town, with the two
switching offices on alternate days. This
situation is often seen in the shared concept
of practice because the individual cost is
less for each of those using the space. Or,
in another type of setting, a single practitioner may maintain several offices, hiring
individuals on either a part-time or full-
time basis to provide semicoverage.

The fourth variable is the type of
patient that will receive services from the
practitioner. With regard to this variable,
the first limitation may be personal. Will
the service be all speech pathology or all
audiology, or, in the case of those clinicians certified in both areas, will both
types of services be provided. Where more
than one individual is involved in a practice, is the practice going to be inter- or
intradisciplinary, and will this be accomplished using only the skills of the two
individuals involved or will consultants be
used? The question of patients' problems is
directly related to the personal skills and
equipment available for the practice.

A second consideration with regard to
the types of patients to be seen may be one
of specific disorders. Does the practitioner
wish to limit his practice primarily to one
kind of disorder (e.g., aphasia, language
disorders, stuttering, structural defects)?
Some practitioners are sufficiently well-

known within a specialty to be able to maintain a full-time practice in that specialty
alone, while others treat various disorders.

Another consideration is that of age;
some clinicians prefer to work only with
school-age children, or some with geriatric
groups.

Setting may present another variable, as
some private practitioners may work only
within a hospital on a contract basis, while
others may work as consultants to schools or
provide a workshop setting for specific disorder groups, such as stutterers.

Limitations of Practice

The majority of practices in this country are probably individual, and the limitations within the individual practice are
those of the clinician's own background and
experience. There is perhaps no other form
of service delivery that is more dependent on
the clinician himself than the indivdual
private practice of speech pathology and/or
audiology. Whether or not one practices
individually and takes responsibility for his
own actions both as a treatment variable and
as a business, the individual must know his
own limitations. The form of his business
may delineate and limit his practice.

Another limitation for a practice is the
growth potential. The community may be able
to support only a very limited number of
patient referrals or services, and this is a
factor in determining the individual practitioner's growth potential both for the type
of service and the geographic area coverage.
In addition, the possibility of adequate
financial return in a given community may be
limited. For example, a small farm community

probably would not support a speech pathologist as well as a large suburban area. This
last restriction probably should be a major
consideration when initiating a private practice.

If the clinician does not wish to limit
his practice, however, or believes that his
skills are such that he can handle a variety
of cases, he may prefer to have a general
practice. In areas where the practioner may
be the only service available to the community, he may serve best through a general
practice.

There are various ways to announce the
opening of a practice, but all must conform
to the Code of Ethics of the American Speech
and Hearing Association. The new practitioner may have personal business cards with his
name, degrees, phone number, address, and
specialty (Fig. 1). Announcements may be
mailed to physicians, psychologists, social
workers, and other practicing speech pathologists and audiologists. These, too, should
list name, degree, specialty, etc. (Fig. 2).
However, experience has demonstrated that
mailing out announcements of the opening of a
practice is costly. While a few may make a
note of the announcement, most will simply
flick the cards into the wastebasket and
forget them.

A more personal approach is to address a
letter to the possible referral source de-
scribing your qualifications (Fig. 3).

The best possible way to announce the
opening of a practice is to make personal
calls on possible referral sources. The new
practitioner should call for an appointment,
be on time, and state his qualifications
briefly and pointedly. If the physician or
other specialist is interested, he will ask

JOHN DOE, Ph.D.
Speech-Language Pathologist

Practice   301 Main
  Restricted to   Houston, Texas
  Children   (713) 678-9101

---

or

JOHN DOE, Ph.D.
Clinical Audiologist

301 Main   (713) 678-9101
Houston, Texas 77027   Hours by
                                  Appointment

FIGURE 1

15

MARY L. SMITH, Ph.D.

and

MARK JOHNSON, Ph.D.

announce the
opening of their
offices for the
practice of

Speech and Language Pathology

and

Clinical Audiology

4291 So. Main Street   (713) 543-2110
Houston, Texas 77004

FIGURE 2

```
          JOHN R. DOE, A.C.S.W.
       3201 West Alabama, Suite 306A
          Houston, Texas 77006
       Telephone:  (713) 661-7421
```

                              May   15,   1972

R. Ray Battin, Psychologist
3931 Essex
Houston, Texas 77027

Dear Dr. Battin:

I am a social worker in private practice
interested in accepting referrals from a
psychologist whose primary area of practice
is psychological testing and evaluation.

My specialties are marital and personal
counseling and casework with children.

Information regarding my background and
experience can be found on the enclosed
curriculum vitae.

If you think that I can be of assistance in
your practice, I would be grateful for a call
from you. I can be reached by telephone at
the number shown above.

Thank you for your consideration.

                         Yours truly,

                         John R. Doe
                         A.C.S.W.

Enc.

                 FIGURE 3

pertinent questions to get further information. Of course, the best source of referral comes from a few successes. A psychiatrist once stated, with regard to referring for evaluation and therapy by a paramedical specialty, "Show us the needs and results and we will overload you with patients." The key is not only in offering a needed service, but then providing an exemplary one.

The decision to enter practice with someone or by oneself has in the past been dictated by each individual's need for independence. Today, it is wise to consider a group practice. Medicine is moving in this direction and certainly so should speech pathology/audiology. Group practice means practice with other speech pathologists and audiologists, with psychologists, with medical social workers, or with various medical disciplines, the most common being the ear, nose, and throat specialist.

Advantages and Disadvantages of Group Private Practice

When an individual becomes part of an organization, some measure of indepencence must be abandoned; thus, group practice is not the form of business chosen by everyone. However, it does provide some special advantages both to the individual within the group and to the public which it serves.

True, group practice does make service delivery easier on the individual practitioner, but its real value lies in its ability to integrate diverse skills in order to better serve the communication-handicapped patient. First, the group practice enables the patient to benefit from the combined experience of qualified individuals representing various types of expertise and all working in the

same place to provide prompt attention to all
of the patient's problems and needs. Second,
the combined financial resources of the group
members permit diagnostic and therapeutic
equipment and skills that an individual may
not be able to afford. Third, the permanence
and continuous functioning of the group
assures the patient that knowledgeable service will be available at all times. Fourth,
this may be the most economical method for
the patient.

The individual within the group practice
is given additional opportunities to improve
himself professionally both by contact with
his associates and attendance at formal
continuing education programs. He is free
from the limiting pressure of a solo practice. He has readily available support and
assurance of consultation from the other
members of the group, as well as a unit
system of records and fee collection which
decreases payment problems.

Some of the disadvantages of group
practice are that a potentially high-earning
specialist might not realize as much income
in a group as in solo practice. Each group
member shares and suffers from the errors of
his associates, as they do from his. Each
member of the group must adhere to the rules
and regulations of the entire group, and this
may limit individualistic expression. Each
group member occasionally will find himself
at odds with the group decision. Finally,
the continuous close relationships involved
may lead to temperamental friction. Third-
party payment, particularly by national
health programs, dictates the type of practice that will be reimbursed for service; in
general, this is a multidisciplined facility
with a medical director.

The authors have had varying experiences
in their independent practices, ranging from

solo practice, which gradually developed into
a multidisciplined practice covering audiology, psychology, psycholinguistics, psycho-
education and speech pathology; solo practice
in audiology/speech pathology in a medical
building with built-in referrals; and, finally, a part-time speech pathology/audiology
practice within a large multidisciplined
medical clinic.

Initial Considerations

Steps in opening one's door to private
practice, then, include proper locale, either
within an established group practice, a group
that is forming, or by oneself. It should
provide easy access for the patients, reasonable distance from the residence of those
served, and adequate parking with little or
no traffic hazards, particularly if young-
sters or invalids are involved. If a solo
practice, it should be close to built-in or
strong referral sources.

Space: Minimum space requirements for
beginning a speech pathology practice include
an office/ therapy room and a comfortable and
attractive waiting room (Fig. 4). Initially,
telephone answering and secretarial services
may be used to handle appointments and typing, thus eliminating the cost of a recep-
tionist/ typist and the space they require.
In a joint practice or partnership, the
waiting room, telephone, and secretarial
costs may be shared.

Non-income-producing space and personnel
are luxuries that the individual going into
private practice can ill afford. In fact,
they can bankrupt even a veteran private
practitioner. Non-income-producing space
includes secretarial areas, office space, and
waiting room space. The practitioner should
evaluate these areas very carefully and allow
for the minimum expenditure needed to provide

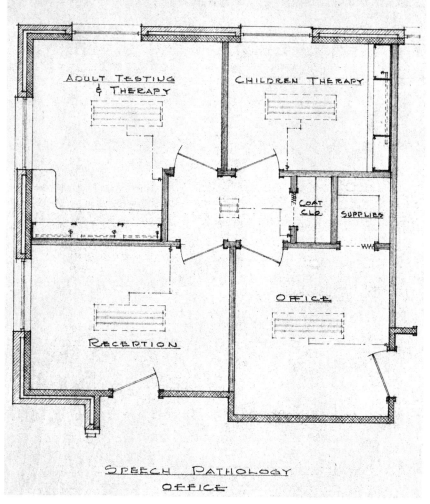

FIGURE 4

adequate comfort and convenience to the
patient. The beginning practitioner should
strongly consider the use of a telephone
answering service and a part-time typist as
opposed to full-time secretarial or office
assistance. Most beginning practitioners can
get by with an answering service and a book-
keeper/typist who can come in only a few
times a month to do simple bookkeeping and
typing. After that, the logical step is to
hire a half-time office employee who can also

21

do bookkeeping, then to hire a full-time receptionist, bookkeeper, and typist.

Minimum requirements for audiology are more expensive and extensive; however, they would also include those of a speech patholo- gist, as far as waiting room and telephone services are concerned.

Location: location of one's practice is critical, as it must be close to several strong referral sources. Acquiring space in a large medical building housing a range of specialities does place one near possible referral sources; however, rents for floor space in such a building will generally be higher than in a smaller professional build- ing. The latter might serve, if strong referral sources have been established prior to opening the service. However, convenience is important to referring physicians, and they will only use a clinic or practitioner outside their immediate environment if there is nothing else available. Frequently a need, formerly unrealized, is established by an audiologist opening a practice; then physicians, particularly otolaryngologists, seeing this need, hire someone to work within their practice for convenience and because they feel there will be financial gain.

Building noise, i.e., air conditioning, blowers, elevators, and street noises, should be carefully reviewed. Often attrative locations have ambient noise levels which are prohibitive to the audiologist. To modify these noises to an acceptable accoustical level is expensive. Since considerable weight is involved with sound rooms, this should be considered when negotiating for space.

Basic Requirements: Opening a private practice in audiology requires a much greater expenditure of funds today than it did to outfit a small office fifteen or more years ago. At that time, one could get by with a single channel "clinical diagnostic audiometer" and add external narrow-band masking and SISI units as it was financially feasible. Today one must enter into practice with a highly sophisticated clinical audiometer. Since hearing aid evaluation is an important part of a clinical audiologist's practice, it is necessary to have not only a two-channel audiometer but also a sound room of adequate size so that speech in noise-free field testing can be done. While ASHA stresses the importance of having a double-walled, two-room suite for audiological testing for any clinic or practice doing extensive hearing testing, it is more logical to set up one's sound room requirements based upon the acoustical environment in which they will be used. This of course suggests that a practitioner should carefully survey the acoustical environment in which he is going to establish his practice prior to purchasing his sound room or rooms. If the structure in which he rents his office space is well built and if the rooms are adaptable to sound treatment, one can get by with a single-walled but large testing room and a treated examiner's room. Today, it is inconceivable to practice without an impedance bridge. Impedance audiometry has come to be an integral part of diagnostic hearing evaluation. It allows the audiologist to analyze middle ear function and disease, to obtain threshold estimates on otherwise untestable infants, and to more comfortably fit amplication to the individual with sensori-neural hearing loss.

In addition to the audiological instrumentation and acoustical rooms, it will be necessary to be equipped with such clinical items as a good otoscope, ear tips of varying sizes, sterilizing equipment, ear molds and ear impression material, battery tester, tubing of varying sizes, etc. Some audiologists are involved in performing electronystagmography, and it is the individual's decision as to whether he wants to provide this diagnostic service to physicians. The cost of instruments is high; space requirements are moderate, but the service does pay for itself if a technician is used to administer the tests. Since ENG's take approximately 1½ to 2 hours, an audiologist's time is too valuable for him to do the actual testing. There is some risk involved, and it would be foolhardy for an audiologist to include ENG's as a part of his practice if he is not in close proximity to physicians.

Once the professional equipment and supply inventory is complete, essential office furniture and supplies should be acquired. At this point, a careful analysis of income-producing versus non-income-producing space and equipment must be made. Income-producing space, of course, refers to the space utilized during patient contact and does not include the audiologist's office (unless he counsels or has patient contact there), the secretary's space, the receptionist's area, or the waiting room. Non-income-producing space should be viewed with a "jaundiced eye." While it would be ideal to have a large, well-appointed waiting room with an office for the secretary/receptionist and a separate work office for the audiologist, it is foolhardy to assume a tremendous financial responsibility at the onset. Psychiatrists seem to have the perfect solution to maintaining a low overhead. Most use an answering service, keep minimal records, and maintain only a small waiting room and a consultation room. Average daily overhead costs for psychiatrists in the Southwest are eight to ten dollars a day. While it would be impossible for an audiologist to keep his

overhead that low, it does suggest that service, not expensive space, is the key to
being adequately compensated for one's time.

CHAPTER II

BUSINESS ASPECTS OF THE PRACTICE

R. Ray Battin, Ph.D. and John L. Boland, Ph.D.

A simple income and outgo system of bookkeeping is all that is necessary, even when a practice grows. It is advisable, however, to have an accountant maintain books and figure depreciation allowance on the purchase of major equipment and furnishings, and usually a CPA is best for this. He will figure the percentage of car expenses that is tax deductible. He can also compute estimated taxes, since income tax will be paid quarterly, based on the estimate for the year. Because there are penalties for misestimating, it is considered "pennywise and pound foolish" for the practitioner to attempt to do this himself, unless he is very skilled in figuring income tax and has some knowledge of tax laws.

Billing

There is a wide choice of billing forms and procedures available to the individual who is entering business. They range from a simple statement form to complicated ledger billing forms, with computerized billing the most comprehensive system.

The beginning practitioner's needs will differ significantly from the requirements of a large medical clinic or a multidisciplinary clinic that provides a wide range of services. When the speech pathologist or audiologist first enters into practice, he will of necessity need to keep his bookkeeping cost

to a minimum. This will determine the type
of ledger system and billing system to be
used. Consultation with an accountant prior
to opening the practice will help in establishing a workable system that is within the
expertise of the practitioner.

Maintaining adequate financial records
which reflect all transactions can be a
tedious task. If the books are set up so
that separate entries must be made on the
statements, ledger books, and day sheets,
plus addressing the envelopes, a tremendous
amount of time and duplication of effort will
be required. A system that requires a minimum of writing and duplication is best. The
Safeguard One-Write System is an example of a
simplified accounting program. This system
requires an accounting board, binder, indexed
tray, patient transaction slips, financial
ledger/statement cards, and day sheets. To
demonstrate the simplicity of this system,
let us say that a patient comes to the audiologist for a routine hearing test. An entry
is made on a patient transaction slip, which
is mounted on the accounting board. The
patient's financial ledger/statement form is
placed between the transaction slip and the
day sheet (a record of charges and receipts).
As the transaction slip is made out indicating services performed and fees, the information is automatically transferred to the
patient's ledger/statement and to the day
sheet. In this way, a single writing at the
time of each transaction (i.e., treatment,
billing, or payment) is all that is required,
thus reducing clerical time.

Initially, hand billing on a monthly
basis by oneself or by a bookkeeping service
or part-time employee is sufficient. Eventually, one may want to convert to computerized
billing. This, of course, depends upon the
size of the practice and the gross income.

The advantages of a computerized billing and accounting service are:

(1)   At-a-glance picture of accounts receivable.

(2)   At-a-glance picture of outstanding accounts, broken down by 30, 60, 90, and 120 days past due.

(3)   Every 30 days a running account as well as a balance sheet and statement of profit and loss.

Collection of Bad Debts

Once an account has become more than 90 days over due, it should be considered high risk. If the practice is large enough to support a receptionist/ typist, she should begin calling on accounts that are 60 days past due and suggest that all future visits be paid at the time of the appointment. Also, an additional amount should be paid on the past-due account until it is paid up to date. The practitioner and his office assistant should then decide whether the individual's payments should remain on a cash basis or whether they can return to a 30-day account.

Lewin (1971), discussing financial accountability of patients of independent practicing psychologists, says:

"Several readers have wondered about methods of collecting long unpaid bills. My immediate reaction is to break 'no pays' into two categories: clients involved in long-term consultation and those who have received brief consultation and/or evaluation services. The importance of lack of payment should be discussed with continuing clients;

it may not only lead to important therapeutic
gains, but can also improve your cash flow.
Repeated lack of response to bills by terminated or brief diagnostic clients is somewhat
different. A note asking for an explanation
and for establishment of a pay schedule is
certainly appropriate. The next step for
many is sending a lawyer's letter threatening
legal action. I am told that this frequently
frightens some chronic debtors into honoring
their debt. As a last resort, collection
agencies are another time-honored technique
for collecting uncollectable balances; however, these companies usually takes one-third
of the amount collected as their fee.

Some practitioners find a large percentage of their billings to be significantly
past due. They, of course, must analyze the
underlying causes of this problem; they can
also take steps to alleviate them by broadening the population they serve. Work with
clients having adequate insurance coverage
can enable the psychological services, and it
assures payment. Work for state and local
social service agencies also guarantees
payment. Many governmental controllers like
to hold on to their monies as long as possible, so payment may be delayed several
months, but be patient--it will arrive."

Establishing Fees

How does a speech pathologist establish
a fee schedule when entering private practice? Charges may be based on an hourly fee
for evaluation time as well as treatment
time, or charges may be made by the test when
doing evaluations. Experience permits one
to estimate the time involved in an evaluation and to set a fee that covers expenses
but is not too punishing to the patient. If
a range is quoted for an intial visit, such

as $30 - $90 based upon time involved, the client (patient) will tend to have a "mental set" in favor of the lower figure. It usually works better to establish an average fee, for example $60, for the initial evaluation, allowing expenses to balance out.

Group therapy charges should be based upon time involved, but at a lower rate than charges for individual treatment. Since additional bookkeeping, record keeping, and report writing costs per hour of treatment time are necessary for group therapy as opposed to individual treatment, the fee for each member in the group should be less than if they received individual care but more than if the hourly treatment fee were divided equally among members of the group.

Several factors need to be taken into consideration when a speech pathologist or audiologist establishes a charge for services. It is necessary to investigate what the practitioner's professional community charges for comparable services. If the practitioner has a master's degree in speech pathology or audiology, then the fee schedule of professionals of comparable training needs to be surveyed. For example, what is the fee schedule for practicing social workers? If the practitioner has doctorate level training, he should investigate the charges of professions, such as psychology, medicine or dentistry, which require the doctorate degree. Realistically, however, the speech pathologist may find himself priced out of business if he tries to build a clientele with fees on a par with those of the psychologist or psychiatrist. In most communities, fees for speech pathology services are measurably lower than those for psychotherapy services. The speech pathologist, therefore, must set fees that reflect his worth and academic expertise, but do not discourage referrals.

A second consideration in setting fees is the cost of doing business. Overhead costs include all of the day-to-day operating expenses: cost of floor space, furniture, telephone, administrative costs, non-income-producing personnel, insurance, office and professional equipment, taxes, and clerical supplies. Furthermore, postage, equipment maintenance, test and therapy supplies, and funds needed for upkeep and replacement of materials and equipment must also be taken into account. The practitioner must project growth needs and constantly refigure replacement costs as these costs change.

Usually, the private practitioner will find that some patients will be able to pay only part of the regular fee and some will be able to pay nothing at all. This loss of income per hour must be accounted for in the total overhead costs. Partial paying or nonpaying patients may be individuals to whom the speech pathologist or audiologist has extended professional courtesy, or they may be individuals who cannot afford to pay, but for whom no other services are available for various reasons. It is the moral and ethical responsibility of every professional person to provide service to some nonpaying patients and to donate a portion of his time to non-income-producing service.

There will always be some patients who simply do not pay. Once a service has been extended, there is no way to take it back, and some people place payment for professional services at the bottom of their payment list. For example, a seminar on budgeting presented recently on local television, discussed the approach used by agencies that assist families in establishing a workable

budget. In determining which bills to pay
first, rent, food, and basic essentials
received priority; payment on repossessables
came second; and payment for services such as
doctor bills was last.

A number of patients will cancel and
others will not show up for appointments.
These losses need to be considered when basic
income needs are figured. These non-filled
appointment times can sometimes be utilized
to return phone calls, write reports, handle
billing chores, or perform other non-income-
producing activities.

Each practitioner must decide how best
to schedule essential non-income-producing
administrative duties, report writing, phone
calls, etc. These are duties that the practitioner cannot ignore. The success of a
practice rests to some extent on the degree
of self-discipline and compulsiveness the
individual has regarding administrative
duties. Many times the private practitioner
finds himself writing reports at home after
his office is closed at the end of the day.

Returning phone calls within a reasonable time is good public relations. It
signifies that the speech pathologist or
audiologist is concerned. Whenever possible,
phone calls from physicians should be
accepted immediately, and patient calls
should be returned the same day. Evening
calls are acceptable to most patients and do
not cut into the practitioner's patient
contact time.

The possibility of losing some work days
due to illnesses must also be considered in
the projected income-versus-overhead cost
equation. One means of figuring anticipated
sick day needs is to allow the same number of

days allowed to salaried employees; generally, this is figured at five days per year.

The final consideration in establishing a fee structure depends upon what the practitioner expects to receive as a reasonable return for his professional work and his investment in the practice. One approach to estimating a reasonable return is to figure the mean salary for an administrator with comparable experience and education in the field of speech pathology. A survey of salary and benefits conducted in 1976 by the Association of Service Programs in Communicative Disorders placed the average salary for a clinic director with three employees between $12,000 and $14,999. Since establishing a practice or business places an individual in an administrative position, it is reasonable to expect a comparable return for one's time. It is also necessary to figure what the return would be on money invested in the practice if the same amount had instead been invested in stocks and bonds. For example, if $20,000 had been used to establish the practice, and figuring 10% as a reasonable return on the invested money, $2,000 for money invested would then be added to overhead costs, etc., when attempting to establish a fee structure. As the speech pathologist's or audiologist's investment and experience grow, adjustments in this formula must be made in order to obtain a reasonable monetary return. Again, using the figures from the 1976 survey, a director of a speech and hearing clinic who has a Ph.D. and who has held the position for more than six years has an average salary of $24,000. If the investment in the practice increased to $100,000 in a comparable time, then the expected return from the private practice should be $34,000.

Using a simple income-outgo accounting system, a hypothetical cost accounting of a private practice for the purpose of establishing fees might indicate the following expenses on a monthly basis. This practice includes the speech pathologist and one employee, a receptionist-secretary.

	C u r r e n t	P e r i o d	A m o u n t	%	P e r i o d	E n d i n g	A m o u n t	%

General Expenses

Accounting and Legal
Auto Expenses
Convention
Depreciation
Donations
Dues-Subscriptions
Entertainment
Payroll Taxes
Other Taxes
Consulting Service
Interest Expenses
Insurance Expenses
Labor and Wages
Licenses and Taxes
Office Expenses
Postage
Rent
Repairs and Maintenance
Equipment Rental
Therapy Supplies
Telephone Expenses
Travel Expenses

     Total General Expenses
     Net Profit or Loss

Assuming that overhead expenses for the month equal $2,200 and adding a reasonable allowance for the practitioner (expected net profit), for example $1,000, costs for the month would be $3,200. Divide this figure by the number of working days in the month (22) and the practitioner has daily costs of $145.46. When this amount is broken down into patient contact time (most clinicians find it difficult to handle more than six hours of direct contact time a day, thus allowing time for telephone calls, report writing, and administrative chores), the required hourly income is $24.24. Since it is necessary to adjust for partial paying, nonpaying, and no-show patients, as well as to anticipate those months which do not provide 22 working days, a minimum charge of $30 to $35 per hour for professional services is required. Since the audiologist could expect to have greater investment and equipment maintenance costs, his per-hour costs should reflect this.

Office Personnel

An independent practitioner, even one in practice by himself, must deal with support personnel as well as professional colleagues. As the practice expands, the practitioner will need to employ such support personnel or staff. These individuals are an extension of the practitioner and the practice, and present his professional image to the public. Care must be taken in selecting office staff, because their interactions with patients may determine whether patients will continue their association with the practitioner. For example, in attempting to schedule an appointment time for a patient who has time limitations, the receptionist-secretary may reflect her frustration in her voice; the patient may interpret this as anger and go elsewhere. Even the person handling the billing reflects the professional image. This person must be accurate, prompt, and courteous. If the patient inquires about his bill, he must be treated courteously and provided with accurate information. If the patient has difficulty meeting his financial obligation, he should be extended some sympathetic understanding and assistance in settling his account.

Most experienced practitioners will agree that the warm, sympathetic voice of a good secretary on the telephone can be one of the most important assets to a practice. The secretary presents the practitioner's professional image to the public when she answers the telephone. She must know a great deal about the employer's professional work because she will usually schedule appointments, answer questions about the practitioner's work, and determine which calls are beyond her scope and should be referred to the practitioner. She should know whether services offered are appropriate for the problem presented. She must also have some knowledge of other referral sources. However, it is also important for the individual answering the telephone and scheduling appointments to know her limitations in answering questions and making referrals.

The women's movement has significantly changed the direction in which women are moving to seek employment; many are less inclined to dedicate themselves to a life-long secretarial career. However, the independent practice depends heavily upon the loyalties of a good secretary. Hence, the traditional attitudes toward the job must be changed, on the part of both the employer and the employee. Dictation equipment, telephone answering equipment, and automatic type-writers can help relieve some of the tedious, "dead-end" chores of the secretary. She can be given a more important role, such as that of a general assistant who is responsible for scheduling, handling minor patient problems that can be dealt with by phone, monitoring testing, assisting in hearing testing of young children, and administering some tests. These are more spophisticated tasks than those usually assigned to a secretary and they require some commitment in terms of time, on the part of both the secretary and the employer. Job stay can be lengthened when the woman continues to see growth potential. Interest in her job and a desire to remain in it can also be accomplished by allowing the secretary-assistant to respond to routine correspondance and to assist in research projects. Appropriate reading material will increase her understanding of the type of clientele seen and ensure that she understands the support she lends to the practice and to the patients. All employees work better if they understand why a task is performed.

As his practice grows, the practitioner may hire additional office personnel. There may, for example, be a bookkeeper, a person to answer the telephone and make appointments, a person to type reports, and perhaps another person to assist in testing and performing other routine office tasks. The number of clerical assistants and their assignments to the various tasks in the office will be determined by the work load.

How can practitioners find efficient office personnel? Secretaries, typists, and other clerical workers can sometimes be found by reading want ads in the local papers. Sometimes the practitioner advertises in the want ads for the clerical help he needs. Clerical workers can sometimes be obtained through employment agencies or through the student employment offices of nearby colleges and universities.

It is hoped that private practitioners will hire office personnel who are honest, capable, loyal, and punctual. Office personnel should be appropriately clean and well groomed, courteous and reasonably attractive physically. Finding such personnel is usually difficult and requires much care and work on the part of the practitioner.

One practitioner uses a short battery of tests for applicants for clerical jobs to learn as much as possible about prospective employees. He wants to learn about the applicant's typing speed and accuracy, and her ability to read, spell, and use the English language correctly. He may give a screening test of personality to screen out persons who are seriously emotionally disturbed. After he has the test data, he interviews the applicant at length and then checks references for further information about the applicant. Even with all these precautions the practitioner will find it difficult to employ and retain effective clerical personnel. Since employing and training new personnel is a time-consuming and expensive process for the practitioner, he will usually find it less expensive in the long run to carefully screen new employees before he hires them. He should reward good employees and be as loyal and courteous to them as he expects them to be to him.

Finally, the use of clerical help and technicians must be reviewed. The beginning practioner needs to ask himself at what point in the development of his practice adding staff will generate more or new practice income. Will this income cover the cost of the new staff? Will adding staff give the practitioner time and energy to develop new

business for the future, and, finally, will
it add to the overall enjoyment of both the
practice and leisure time. Most speech
pathologists and audiologists lack managerial
training and may underestimate the drain on
time and energy.

Vacation and Convention Attendance

Absences from the office can be expensive for the speech pathologist or audiologist. Almost all office expenses continue
during the practioner's absence--secretaries,
salaries, heat, light, telephone, and all of
the many other expenses of operating an
office. In addition, the practitioner loses
the income he would have made during the
office hours.

It is evident, however, that the practitioner needs vacations to rest and to replen-
ish his strength. From time to time, he also
needs professional stimulation that he can
receive in attending conventions, seminars,
and workshops. The needs of the practitioner
for vacations and for professional stimulation must be balanced against his financial
needs and the needs of his patients.

The practitioner must carefully consider
the needs of his patients and his referral
sources when planning his vacations and other
absences from his office. Some practitioners
find it advantageous to take vacations at the
same time each year. Patients and referral
sources learn that the practitioner will be
on vacation during all of August or he will
take a week's vacation in June and another
week in December. Patients and referral
sources can learn to anticipate the vacations
of the professional and plan their own schedules accordingly.

Professional meetings can often be planned in advance also. Professional meetings attended by private practioners are usually short, are held on weekends, are held in sites that are easily available by airplane. The practitioner should, as much as possible, coordinate his absences with the needs of referring physicians and other referral sources. Vacations can often be scheduled during a time of the year when the practitioner's professional activities are relatively slow.

It is usually difficult or impossible for the practicing speech pathologist to have a substitute see his patients during his absence. The relationship between the patient and the speech pathologist is usually a close one, and substitutes are not usually acceptable to the patient. The audiologist, on the other hand, may be able to arrange to have another audiologist do routine audiological evaluations during his absence. The needs of the referring physicians for immediate audiological evaluations can thus be met and the substitute audiologist can arrange for the patient to be seen again by the regular practitioner if the case proves to be a difficult one or one with which the substitute audiologist does not feel comfortable or familiar.

The practitioner's anticipated absences should be discussed with his patient as early as possible. The practitioner can encourage the patient to talk about his feelings about the practitioner's anticipated absences-- sometimes patients feel anger, abandonment, fright, or have other feelings about the practitioner's anticipated absences. He should be encouraged to express these feelings before the absence and when the practitioner returns.

Absences should be kept to a minimum.
If the practitioner wants the patient to feel
that treatment twice a week is important,
offering the treatment twice a week must be
important to the practitioner. If the practitioner is often absent, the patient can
easily get the feeling that consistent treatment is not important to the practitioner or
to the patient, and the patient then starts
being absent himself.

But with all these precautions, it is
obviously important that the professional
engage in continuing education to improve and
sharpen his professional skills. Private
practitioners often feel lonely and isolated,
so it is vital to them to have opportunities
to associate with their professional peers.

What Price Growth?

As the individual's practice expands, he
is faced with acquiring staff or adding to
his present staff. He must ask himself,
"What price growth?" Most independent practitioners in speech pathology and audiology
regard growth as an unquestionably important
goal. Growth in services extended; growth in
space, equipment, and staff size; and growth
in earnings are all sought after as the
ultimate goal of a developing practice.
Growth will bring a lot of changes and,
sometimes, disaster to an independent practice. Before growth for growth's sake is
blindly pursued, the practitioner must evaluate his increasing administrative and managerial duties, for he will have less and less
time to spend in the clinical role.

A practice that grows successfully will
pass through several distinct phases. The
first phase generally consists of a single-
person practice with efforts centered on

promotion and provision of service. Organization is generally informal and the practitioner and any part-time or full-time employees tend to be "jacks of all trades" rather than specialists. The practitioner may schedule his own appointments, send out his own bills, and do the typing at first, gradually turning these duties over as employees are brought in to assist the practice. Decisions regarding income, outgo, and scheduling are made quickly and are based upon an intimate knowledge of time and budget.

As the practice begins to grow, more organization and control procedures become necessary. Specialized business expertise, such as specialized knowledge in financial and business management, becomes necessary. The owner/practitioner is no longer able to maintain personal supervision of all aspects of maintaining and operating the practice, and a professional business manager may be brought in on either a consultative or full-time basis.

As additional professional help is brought into the practice, the original owner/practitioner must share authority in order to maintain growth. He will find himself becoming involved only in "problem areas" of management. While he still maintains central control and identity of the practice, he has little involvement in managing the day-to-day workings of the practice.

As diversification of the practice occurs and different specialities are brought together, management of the practice may be shared, thus leading to a lack of coordination and direction. Controls regarding yearly budgets for equipment, maintenance expenditures, and salaries will need to be instigated. Increased control procedures become cumbersome, and there is often a loss of personal interest and identity with the practice. At this stage in development, the originator of the practice will find himself removed from its day-to-day operation, and will receive complaints and information only through formalized channels. He may find that he has lost flexibility, creativity, motivation, and visibility; in fact, he may have lost his "raison d'être."

Considerations for Retirement and Investments

The private practicing speech pathologist/audiologist will find that he is engaged in a business as well in professional practice. He has the satisfactions of a professional person but he also has problems and opportunities that businessmen have.

Very early in his practice he will be confronted with questions about how his business is to be organized. Does he want to be a solo practitioner or a partner with other practitioners, or does he want to incorporate his practice? There are advantages and disadvantages to each way of practicing. The solo practitioner can have a minimum number of employees and can set his own schedule and conduct his practice with a maximum degree of independence. He may decide, for example, to teach half time and practice speech pathology half time. The next year he may decide to arrange his time in some other way. A partnership or corporation is more formal, however, and requires the practitioner to project the use of his professional time more specifically before he enters into such an arrangement.

The type of business arranagement he makes will often be determined, to a great extent, by income tax considerations.

Speech pathology/audiology training programs usually contain little information about the business aspects of practice and about estate building and estate planning. Also, there seems to be little correlation between a practitioner's professional competence and his business sense. If anything, there may be an inverse relationship. As a result, there are many persons who make their living by selling questionable insurance, questionable investments, and questionable advice to private practitioners.

The prudent private practitioner, therefore will seek the best advice he can find. A competent attorney and a competent accountant who are familiar with his practice can advise him about the tax consequences of his business arrangement, about retirement plans, estate building, estate planning, and many other problems that he will encounter.

The speech pathologist/audiologist who is an employee of a university, a clinic, or a hospital usually participates in a retirement plan that has been set up by the employing institution. The private practitioner has no such built in retirement plan. Very early in his practice, he must consider how he can invest the money he makes above operating expenses so that he will be able to retire someday.

The private practitioner can invest his surplus funds in many ways. Many business management consultants advise businessmen to invest as much as possible in their own businesses. In theory, investing in one's own business should yield greater dividends than investing in other businesses. There is

a limit, however, to the amount of money a
practitioner can invest in his own business,
so plans to invest in other ways need to be
considered.

Surplus funds can be invested in land,
buildings, houses, stocks and bonds, an-
tiques, books, etc. The multiplicity of
investment opportunities is so bewildering
that the young practitioner often has difficulty choosing the investment opportunities
that would be best for him in his particular
situation.

Again, income tax consequences play an
important part in decisions about how the
practitioner should invest his surplus funds.

It is possible to invest money received
during one's high-income years and defer
paying income tax until one retires and his
income declines. The practitioner may have
to pay 25% to 50% income tax on his income
during his high-income years. Later when he
becomes semiretired or retired, his income,
as well as his income tax, may be much less.
There are ways in which he can save some of
the funds he earns during his high-income
years and postpone paying income tax until he
is ready to retire.

The direct purchase of annuities in bond
purchase plans has been approved by the
internal revenue code as a way of saving
money and postponing income tax. Other ways
have been devised. Some of these are described in the following paragraphs.

The Individual Retirement Savings Plan
(IRA) is one of the simpler plans approved by
the Internal Revenue Service by which a
practitioner can save money each year and
postpone the paying of income tax until he
retires. A self-employed individual can save

a maximum of $1,500 each year in an IRA, and a married individual with an unemployed spouse can deduct up to $1,750 each year for contributions to separate IRA's for himself and his spouse, up to a maximum of 15% of his earned income. IRA funds may be invested in a number of ways which have been approved by the IRS. The invested funds must be distributed to the practitioner between the ages of 59½ and 79½. Ordinary income tax is then paid on the proceeds of the plan. It is important to note that the practitioner's employees need not participate in the practitioner's IRA plan.

Much greater annual contributions may be made by the practitioner to an HR-10 Keogh Plan. The practitioner may contribute 15% of his earned income, not to exceed $7,500, each year to his Keogh Plan. The first $100,000 of earnings may be taken into account under this plan.

Generally, anybody who is self-employed and has earnings from personal services which he renders can have a Keogh Plan. An important consideration concerning the Keogh Plan is that all the practitioner's employees who have worked for him for three years or more must be covered if the practitioner wants to cover himself. A practitioner who contributes 10% of his income to the Keogh Plan, therefore, must contribute 10% of the salaries of his employees to the plan also.

The added expense of covering other employees often costs more than the tax benefits that the practitioner gets for himself under the plan. On the other hand, a practitioner in a high tax bracket may be able to come out ahead, even though he has to cover his employees. The only way to be sure that it is profitable for a proprietor to have such a plan is to work out the projected figures.

Management consultants usually advise a practitioner to consider the corporate form of business practice when his taxable earnings reach the $25,000 to $50,000 bracket. There are advantages and disadvantages to incorporating one's practice, so the pros and cons of such a strategy need to be carefully examined.

Many professional persons across the country--architects, accountants, dentists, physicians, and attorneys--are turning their practices into corporations. Sometimes the practitioner may form the same kind of corporation as any other business. Some states, however, specify that certain types of professionals who incorporate must form "professional corporations." Only by consulting the laws of your state can you decide whether you may incorporate as any other business or whether you must incorporate as a professional corporation.

The key difference between a corportion and self-employment is that when he incorporates, the professional is a "common law employee" of his own corporation. As a result, the individual is eligible for a wide range of personal financial benefits available only to employees.

Some of the advantages to incorporation are the following: (1) A corporation may adopt a qualified profit-sharing and pension plan which permits the practitioner to invest up to 25% of his income in tax-deferred investments. Thus, the provisions covering contributions to corporate pension plans and profit-sharing plans are more liberal than those covering contribution plans for the self-employed. (2) The corporation may provide all of its employees with group term life insurance, the first $50,000 of which is not considered as taxable income to the employee. (3) The corporation may provide all or a portion of its employees with medical insurance, medical reimbursement payments, and wage continuation payments or insurance in the case of disability.

It must be remembered that all employees must participate in a corporate pension plan or profit-sharing plan. The cost of including all of his employees under such a plan must be carefully considered by the practitioner.

Major drawbacks to incorporation are the additional red tape and bureaucratic entanglements involved in operating the practice. Most corporations and professional corporations are required to organize under state laws, issue stock certificates, prepare annual reports, and pay filing fees.

The practitioner considering incorporation should review the matter thoroughly with his accountant and attorney. This complex area requires a great deal of extra knowledge. The best advice is to get all the competent help you can.

The material above concerning the IRA, the Keogh Plan, incorportion, profit-sharing, and pension plans associated with the corporation is incomplete. More detailed information may be obtained from banks, insurance companies, attorneys, and accountants. Many other ways of postponing the payment of income taxes on current income also have been devised.

It is well to remember that some management consultants regard the retirement plans for the self-employed described above as mistakes. The argue that the value of money is going down and income taxes are increasing, historically. Thus, the $100 you invest today will be worth much less in 20 years and the income tax rate may be much higher at that time. These consultants advise young practitioners to pay the income tax on the money they make now and invest their surplus funds in land, stocks, or other investments that will, in theory, increase in value over the years.

Excellent information about retirement plans can be found in the May 31, 1976, issue of <u>Medical Economics</u> as well as the January 1978 issue of <u>Psychotherapy Finances</u>. The later is a monthly newletter which provides up-to-date information on third-party payment, billing, pension plans, and other business news pertinent to the private practitioner.

REFERENCES

Lewin MH: Towards a bolder model, Professional Psychology, Winter, New York, 1971, p.
83

Lewin M: Successful Professional Practice,
New York, Capital Professional Development
Institute, 1978

CHAPTER III

A CONSIDERATION OF OUTPATIENT SPEECH
AND
LANGUAGE PATHOLOGY SERVICES UNDER MEDICARE

H. Aubrey Feiwell, M.A.

Private practioners can work independently on their own recognizance. They can
do contracts, disseminate services on referral, or provide services as a rehabilitation
agency. The private practitioner who opts to
work independently may submit billings on the
basis of a prudent buyer concept; however, a
rehabilitation agency must offer services on
a reasonable cost basis.

On June 21, 1976, regulations specifying
conditions of participation for clinics,
rehabilitation agencies, and public health
agencies as providers of outpatient speech
pathology services under Medicare Part B
became effective. The regulations were
promulgated by the Social Security Administration to implement the 1972 amendments
(Public Law 92-603) to section 1861(p) of the
Social Security Act.

The Act applies the conditions for
outpatient physical therapy services to
outpatient speech pathology services. Outpatient physical therapy services are defined
in the law as services furnished by a provider of services, (i.e., hospital, skilled
nursing facility, home health agency) a
clinic, rehabilitation agency, or public
health agency, or by others under an arrangement with and under the supervision of such
provider, clinic rehabilitation agency, or
public health agency to an individual as an

outpatient. The Medicare beneficiary served
by an outpatient facility must be under the
care of a physician who prescribes the type,
amount, and duration of services to be furnished, and who reviews the plan of treatment
at 30-day intervals, i.e., recertification.

There are three types of businesses
which may become certified Medicare providers
of outpatient speech pathology services:
public health agencies, rehabilitation agencies, and clinics. The term "clinic" is used
to identify a facility established primarily
for the provision of outpatient physicians'
services. Under the clinic certificiation
option, two physicians must be on staff, and
there are dollar restrictions in terms of
treating the patient.

An individual in private practice would
be categorized under the regulations as a
"rehabilitation agency." A "rehabilitation
agency" is defined as: "An agency which
provides an integrated multidisciplinary
program designed to upgrade the physical
function of handicapped, disabled individuals
by bringing together as a team specialized
rehabilitation personnel. At a minimum, a
rehabilitation agency must provide physical
therapy or speech pathology services, and a
rehabilitation program which, in addition to
physical therapy or speech pathology services, includes social or vocational adjustment services." A "public health agency" is
an official agency established by a state or
local government.

Conditions of Participation

To participate as a provider of services, the rehabilitation agency or clinic is
required to satisfy certain requirements
relating to clinical records, policies govern-

ing the services provided, state or local licensure, plans of care for each patient established and periodically reviewed by a physician, adequate facilities and equipment to carry out a program of treatment, and a sufficient number of properly qualified personnel. Each state department of public health assists the Social Security Administration (SSA) in determining whether clinics and agencies in each state meet the Medicare requirements.

After the state department of public health receives the Request to Establish Eligibility (Form SSA-1856), it will schedule a survey of the organization. The organization will be informed of the date a survey team will come to interview and carry out procedures necessary to determine whether the organization meets the requirements of participation. In addition to speech pathology, an additional professional service must be offered by the rehabilitation agency. In some instances, the second service which qualifies the team as a rehabilitation agency will be non-reimbursable. For example, in the case of clinical psychology, the Medicare program provides for reimbursement up to $100 annually for each patient, for diagnosis only. If a physician refers a patient to the agency for psychological testing and treatment, the agency, in order to meet the conditions of participation, must offer the services indicated by the patient's diagnosis and provide treatment that is medically necessary. The Department of Health, Education, and Welfare will notify each organization that does not meet the Conditions of Participation and which cannot, therefore, participate in the Medicare program.

The Department of Health, Education, and Welfare, under the Social Security Administration, has printed Medicare Provider Reim-

bursement Manuals for the individual who
provides services under the Medicare law.
These Manuals are referred to as "HIM" and
have numbers which signify specific types of
information. The manual provides guidelines
and policies to implement the Medicare regulations so that the individual can understand
the principals that the agency follows for
determining the reasonable cost of provider
services. The private practitioner in speech
pathology and audiology does not have specific guidelines provided for him, and, for the
most part, we have been lumped under the
guideline manual provided for outpatient
physical therapy. Consider that the guidelines for speech pathology have been attempted to be processed under and in accordance with the outpatient physical therapy
guidelines and subsequently do not always fit
specifically. In this case, because the
provider guidelines have not been specifically outlined, the private practitioner in
speech pathology is faced with many new and
different problems for which the federal
government has not mandated specific procedures. Therefore, the processing of claims
is in formative stages.

At present, Medicare Part B carriers are
responsible for making payments on a reasonable cost basis to participating clinic
providers. The concept of "reasonable cost"
is subject to interpretation. If the organization is found to be eligible, a representative of the department will countersign the
agreement; reimbursement for services rendered to Medicare beneficiaries can be made
as of the effective date of the agreement.

Information Regarding the Terms
of Reimbursement

Medicare part B carriers are responsible for making payments on a reasonable cost basis to participating clinic providers. Jurisdiction for handling clinic providers is the same as that established for other Part B services, i.e., all clinic providers are serviced by that carrier. Payments to rehabilitation and public health agencies approved for the purpose of rendering outpatient physical therapy and/or outpatient speech pathology services are made by Part A intermediaries. The agencies may elect to deal directly with SSA (direct reimbursement). The intermediary selection is subject to SSA approval on the basis that it is in the interest of efficient and effective program administration. The Social Security Administration has decreed that private insurance companies will act as insurers under the Medicare Program. In some states this may be Blue Cross and Blue Shield, Travelers Insurance Company, Mutual Benefit of Omaha, and so forth. All of these insurers are designated as "fiscal intermediaries" and/or "carriers."

Under the 1967 amendments to the Social Security Act, approved clinics, rehabilitation agencies, and public health agencies may receive reimbursement for 80 percent of the reasonable cost of outpatient physical therapy and speech pathology services. The remaining 20 percent of charges would be payable by the patient. These services are reimbursable (apart from services rendered by a home health agency) under the medical insurance program, after the annual $60.00 medical insurance deductible has been incurred by the beneficiary.

The cost reimbursement policy would permit clinics, rehabilitation agencies, and public health agencies to receive reasonable cost reimbursement for outpatient physical therapy and speech pathology services rendered. The principles of reimbursement applicable to hospitals, skilled nursing facilities, and home health agencies that participate in the Medicare program are also applicable to providers of outpatient physical therapy and/or speech pathology services.

For cost reporting purposes, the program requires submission of annual reports covering a 12-month period of operations based upon the provider's established cost reporting period. The cost data submitted must be based on the accrual basis of accounting, which is recognized as the most accurate basis for determining costs as based on what you charge and not necessarily on what you collect. For example, if you treated a patient at a cost of $35.00 a session and you saw this patient three times a week, at a total cost of $105.00 a week, and you failed to collect the monies either from the patient's carrier or the patient, the entry in your books would be valid and taxable until such time as you are able to establish it as a bad debt and reverse the charges. This is in contrast to a cash basis of accounting in which you pay taxes on monies which you have actually received and deposited. Public health agencies that operate on a cash basis of accounting may submit their annual cost reports on this basis, with the exception of capital expenditures. Extensive cost statement forms for calculation of the reimbursable cost of physical therapy and speech pathology services are issued upon approval of a provider number and acceptance of the agency or clinic by the fiscal intermediary.

The cost report is due at the intermediary's office on or before the last day of
the third month following the close of that
period (Section 2413, Provider Reimbursement
Manual). If a complete cost report is not
received by the deadline, the intermediary
will reduce the agency's interim payment
(Section 2409, Provider Reimbursement Manual). This reduction would be 31 days following the last day available for timely
submission of the cost report.

Worksheets or schedules required by law
must be filled in in their entirety on specific forms required by the state and/or federal governments. The agency still has the
option of submitting a copy of its audited
financial statement in lieu of the aforemen-
tioned worksheets or schedules, if the statement contains the necessary detail. However,
one or the other must accompany the complete
Medicare cost report. Failure to meet this
requirement will result in a reduction in
interim rates following the agency's cost
report due date. All worksheets and schedules that are not applicable must be so
marked and returned with the completed cost
report.

When extenuating circumstances exist, an
extension not to exceed one month can be
granted. A written request for such an
extension, with reasons, must be submitted
before the 90-day due date.

Practical Considerations

The private practitioner of speech
pathology needs to ascertain the appropriate-
ness, in terms of his practice, of applying
for a provider number (rehabilitation agency
status). Good and adequate decisions are
usually made on the basis of available facts;

therefore, this decision will not be an easy one, due to the paucity of functional data. The conditions of participation for this program are embryonic, and in need of patience, cooperation, and mutually conceived guidelines.

Prior to applying for rehabilitation agency status, it is recommended that contact be made with the proposed fiscal intermediary to determine its readiness for speech pathology in terms of billing procedures and degree of rehabilitation orientation. A fiscal intermediary poorly oriented to rehabilitation might reject many or all of the agency's claims.

The following questions are posed to assist the prospective practitioner in determining the merits of pursuing rehabilitation agency status:

1. How will rehabilitation agency status help me serve my patients better?

2. Will the acquisition of a provider number enable me to serve more of the geriatric population?

3. If the answer to #2 is "Yes," am I eager to increase the geriatric patient load?

4. What percentage of my present patient load is made up of persons who are younger than 65 years of age but who have been disabled for a period of 24 months or longer?

5. Do I think that rehabilitation agency status will assist me in obtaining additional outpatient coverage from other carriers?

6. Do I want to enlarge my office practice to include the treatment of various types of speech and language disorders on an outpatient basis (these could be patients who are being treated currently at a hospital on an outpatient basis because treatment is not a covered benefit at the office)?

7. How will rehabilitation agency status affect the composition and/or character of the total patient load?

8. Am I desirous of such a change?

9. Am I willing to orient my ideas to new conditions?

10. Do I think I might be relinquishing some of my professional freedom in and control over my practice?

If the prospective applicant decides that the acquisition of rehabilitation agency status is desirable, he or she should be equipped to handle the increase in clerical, work. Some examples of this are:

1. Initial site visit by the department of public health (survey team).

2. Compliance with "deficiencies."

3. 0719 Blue Cross, Speech and Hearing Pathology Information; or 4145 The Travelers Insurance Companies, Speech Pathology and Audiology Plan of Treatment.

4. Daily Progress Reports (see Figure 1).

5. Patient Care Form (see Figure 2).

6. Speech and Language Pathology Services, Treatment Plan, and Recertification (see Figure 3).

7. Utilization Review Form (see Figure 4).

8. Form SSA-1483, Provider Billing for Medical and Other Health Services.

9. Form SSA-2088, Physical Therapy Provider Statement of Reimbursable Cost for Outpatient Physical Therapy Services Furnished by Rehabilitation Agencies, Clinics, and Public Health Agencies.

This clerical and accounting work is in addition to the normal and familiar documentation of initial speech and language pathology evaluation, re-evaluation, and other diagnostic reporting.

A complete discussion of "clinic" status has not been included in this chapter, because the author does not consider it to be an appropriate alternative for speech and language pathologists.

APPENDIX

CHAPTER III

NAME:

P.C. #:

SNF:

SNF #:

H. AUBREY FEIWELL, M.A.,   TELEPHONE
SPEECH AND LANGUAGE PATHOLOGY, P.C. AC 313-642-4550

SPEECH AND LANGUAGE PATHOLOGY PROGRESS

DATE		INITIALS

64

FIGURE 1

H. AUBREY FEIWELL, M.A., SPEECH & LANGUAGE PATHOLOGY, P.C.

PATIENT CARE FORM

Name _____   Address _____

Record No. _____

HIC/BC-BS No. _____

Patient Care Plan
(Explain details of care, treatments, teaching, habits, preferences, and goals.)

Check if Pertinent:

DISABILITIES	BEHAVIOR	IMPAIRMENTS	COMMUNICATION
☐ Amputation	☐ Alert	☐ Speech	☐ Can Write
☐ Paralysis	☐ Forgetful	☐ Hearing	☐ Talks
☐ Contractures	☐ Noisy	☐ Vision	☐ Understands Speaking
☐ Decubitus	☐ Confused	☐ Sensation	☐ Understands English
☐ Other	☐ Withdrawn	☐ Other	☐ If no, Other Language?
	☐ Wanders		☐ Reads
	☐ Other		☐ Non-Verbal

REQUIRES

☐ Colostomy Care   ☐ Cane   ☐ Crutches   ☐ Walker   ☐ Wheelchair

☐ Dentures   ☐ Eye Glasses   ☐ Hearing Aid   ☐ Prosthesis   ☐ Side Rails

☐ Other

<u>SOCIAL INFORMATION</u> (including patient's personality, attitude toward illness and family constellation and inter-relationships):

TREATMENT (Speech, Psychology, Other _____)

_____
Signature of Professional

Telephone _____   Date _____

FIGURE 2

67

H. AUBREY FEIWELL, M.A., SPEECH AND LANGUAGE PATHOLOGY, P.C.

SPEECH AND LANGUAGE PATHOLOGY SERVICES, TREATMENT PLAN, AND RECERTIFICATION

Patient's Number _____

Patient's Name _____ BD: _____ AGE _____

Address _____

Phone _____ HIC/BC-BS# _____

Date Patient Evaluated _____ Soc. Sec. # _____

Diagnosis: _____

_____

_____

Date of onset of illness _____
(Date of surgery, if any)

Anticipated goals: _____

_____

_____

If this is a continuation of treatment previously authorized, is there a noticeable improvement in patient's condition: _____

I certify/re-certify that the above-named patient is under my care and that the speech and language pathology treatments ordered for this patient are medically necessary.

Date: _____

_____
Signature of Physician

_____
Name of Physician

FIGURE 3

H. AUBREY FEIWELL, M.A., SPEECH & LANGUAGE PATHOLOGY, P.C.

UTILIZATION REVIEW FORM

NAME _____

(This section to be completed by person responsible for medical records)

(This section to be completed by Speech & Language Pathologist) **Please circle as appropriate.**

1. _____
   (Rehabilitation Agency — Name, Address, City, State & Zip Code)

2. _____ 3. _____ 4. _____ 5. _____
   (Patient Identification No.) (Age) (Sex) (1st Treatment Date)

6. Amitted to Skilled Nursing Facility from: (please circle)

   a) Acute Hospital _____ Number of Days Stay _____

   b) Home After Hospital Discharge Number of Days Home _____

   c) Another SNF _____ Number of Days Stay _____

7. Primary Diagnosis: _____

   (Other) _____

8. Present Diagnosis: _____
   _____

9. Has/is patient receiving treatment: Yes ___ No ___ a)Speech ___ b)Other ___

   c)Number of treatments _____ d)Date of last Treatment _____

10. Date of last visit by attending physician _____

11. Attending physician's recommendations for continued care (please summarize) _____
    _____

13. Mental Status: a) alert _____ b) confused _____ c)forgetful _____

14. Behavior: a) cooperative b) belligerent c)noisy d) senile
    e) withdrawn f) socializes

15. Impairments: a) aphasic   b)hearing   c) speech
                  d) sensation e) vision   f) language

16. Care Status: a) independent   b) dependent

    (Please use code for items below:
    I=Independent   D=Dependent

    Ambulation: ☐ alone   ☐ attendant   ☐ cane
                 ☐ walkerette ☐ wheelchair

    Feeding: ☐ fork   ☐ spoon   ☐ knife
              ☐ glass ☐ cup   ☐ fed

17. Patient's rehabilitative condition in terms of _____ has:
    improved _____ deteriorated _____ remained static _____ since admission to this SNF _____ since last review _____ .

18. _____
    (Signature of professional making this report — Date of report)
    Space is provided on back for information of other professional personnel if it is felt desirable to include.

19. Supplemental information from rehabilitation specialists consultants summarized: _____
    _____

12. Days in this SNF to current date _____ Date of last review _____

Date _____

Name or signature
of attending physician _____

UTILIZATION REVIEW COMMITTEE CHECK LIST
(To be completed by reviewing physician)

Check as appropriate with explanatory note if necessary:

1. Was admission to treatment necessary? If NO indicate other
facility or agency that could have provided services.　Yes ☐　No ☐

Comment: _____

2. Could length of treatment have been shortened without
adverse effect to patient?　Yes ☐　No ☐

Comment: _____

3. Was appropriate use made of other rehabilitation services
to improve quality of care?　Yes ☐　No ☐

Comment: _____

4. Are additional services necessary?　Yes ☐　No ☐

a) If YES please indicate type _____

5. Is further treatment recommended?　Yes ☐　No ☐

If YES complete the following:

a) Reason for continued treatment _____

b) Date of next review _____

Form No. HAFPC : 42877-1

If NO complete the following: (UR Chairman see below)

Reason discontinuation is recommended _____

d) Recommendation for other type treatment (if any) _____

6. Date of review _____

Signature or code number
of reviewing physician _____

7. Date _____

Signature or code number
of the U.R.C. Chairman _____

8. TO BE COMPLETED IF CONTINUED TREATMENT IS
DISAPPROVED:
Letter sent to following:
a) attending physician _____ Date _____
b) facility _____ Date _____
c) responsible party _____ Date _____

FOR USE OF REHABILITATION AGENCY ONLY

Sent to U.R.C. on _____ Returned after review on _____

Decision _____

Disposition and/or date of new review _____

FIGURE 4

CHAPTER IV

FORENSIC SPEECH PATHOLOGY

Donna R. Fox, Ph.D.

The question of ethics has become one of interest to the private practitioner in recent years because of more personal involvement in subsequent decisions. Ethics are defined by Webster as a moral code of good and bad. This code can be applied to the individual's personal behavior code as well as to his professional code. Conflict ensues when guidelines are not clearly defined. The speech pathologist's professional behavior is defined in the American Speech and Hearing Association's Code of Ethics, but even here conflict occurs between what is good for the consumer and what is good for the profession. When certain standards are not met by members of a society (cultural or professional), then behavioral guidelines are attached to some legal process and adherence by all members of that society is mandatory.

When a patient contacts a professional, an unwritten contract goes into effect. Because of some thing or problem, a patient seeks professional guidance to some solution or affirmative goal. The contract then becomes binding on the professional to provide the best professional service of which he is capable. However, the patient may or may not accept or follow up on the advised direction. The contract does not become binding upon the patient until he enters into treatment. The professional must remember that he is obligated to give the most reasonable and sound advice he can, while the pa-

tient is not bound to accept. He is bound,
however, to pay his bill.

The speech pathologist may be involved
with the legal profession in two major roles:
as an expert witness or as the recipient of a
legal suit for injury, malpractice, or libel.
For the speech pathologist in private practice, some knowledge of the state laws regarding individual and/or corporate responsibility is essential. As an expert witness, the
speech pathologist is most often involved in
cases concerning custody of minors, personal
injury, and competency.

The following was originally published
by the Bulletin of the American Academy of
Private Practice in Speech Pathology and
Audiology for members, and is included here
by the author as originally published.

When a speech pathologist
receives academic training in this
behavioral speciality little or no
emphasis is placed on his position
with the law or on the possibility
that this specialized training may
place him in the position of
"expert witness." An expert witness is defined by Liebenson and
Wepman as:

"one who possesses special
knowledge and experience on
matters and issues in a
lawsuit. This would include
all issues involving scientific or other special knowledge. His function in court
is to assist the jurors in
arriving at a correct con-
clusion upon matters that are
not familiar to their every-

day experiences so that they may arrive at an intelligent understanding of the issues that must be decided."

The expert witness differs from other types of witnesses in that he is allowed to answer questions of opinion regarding his specialty. More and more often the possessors of specialized knowledge of speech and hearing are being called upon to provide testimony in courts of law and quasi-judicial proceedings. Such testimony can be provided in person and through written reports but in either case the courtroom experience can often be devastating to the unprepared and the uninformed.

A speech pathologist or audiologist acting as a consultant on a specific case is not unusual, but when he is called into a case as a consultant in which his opinion will have a bearing on the outcome of a lawsuit he assumes an entirely different role. This average person sees court as time-consuming, objectionable, and something to be avoided. However, knowledge of some points of information concerning the position and behavior of the speech pathologist/audiologist in a courtroom proceeding can be helpful to the overall presentation of his findings.

State laws vary and each speech-language pathologist/audiologist should have some information concerning the availability of his records and himself to the court. In some states, records can be subpoenaed from anyone including physicians at an instant's notice. There is no such thing as privileged communication. This is also true of the individual himself. Records of an individual case should be thorough and unbiased, with test procedures, results, and techniques employed reported accurately. In addition, records should indicate the separation of scientific fact from interpretation and opinion. Don't put anything into a record you don't want to read to a juror.

If you are ordered to appear in court, failure to do so can have grim results. In some states this can result not only in a fine but also in imprisonment. However, you may only be asked by either party in a law case to appear and you can choose whether or not you wish to do so. Only if you are subpoenaed must you appear. Types of cases in which expert witnesses are called can be either civil or criminal but most often the personal injury and divorce suits in which the custody of a child is a question, may call for expert witness testimony. In any case any speech pathologist/audiologist who is involved in private practice or as a consultant in any way to public or private agencies would be wise to be well informed on the laws of the state which pertain to record availability, licensing, and qualifications of expert witnesses.

If you are asked to appear as an expert witness you should be prepared to indicate your education, background and experience. "Experience is the essential legal ingredient of competence to give an expert opinion (Liebenson and Wepman, 1964)." In most states this attitude holds. For the most part in the field of speech pathology and audiology the expert witness would be expected to indicate academic and experience competency. He may hold a Ph.D. degree, be a member of ASHA, and hold Certification of Clinical Competency, be licensed or certified by a state agency or meet local specified regulations. More and more the Certificate of Clinical Competence is being requested not only in cases in court of law but by insurance companies, hospitals, and other public agencies as a criterion for expertise. You can expect to be asked about membership in other organizations, any kind of licensing or any publications or honors in the field which would qualify you as an expert. In addition, you may be asked about the kind of testing equipment that is usual for a speech pathologist and audiologist. The use of examples and clarification of procedures is of utmost importance. Any clinician seeing a client under any circumstances can be summoned to testify when some medico-legal issue occurs.

Conduct in the courtroom can have varying effect upon the jurors. You should be pleasant,

precise, and punctual. Language
and terminology that can be defined
and understood easily seems to be
most helpful. Too often the expert
witness uses terminology within his
own field which is not understood
by other members of the courtroom
and this may lead to misunderstand-
ing. In most cases you are permitted to use notes and may ask to
refresh your memory from time to
time regarding certain detailed
aspects of the case; however, it is
best to testify in a direct,
straight forward manner in answering questions rather than to read
prepared answers. Most important
for you to remember is the reason
you have been asked to appear as a
witness. You are there because you
have some information or special
knowledge which is pertinent to the
issues in a given case. The information you possess may be negative
or positive, but it has been deemed
essential to prove or disprove an
issue. Your conduct and presentation of that information can
affect the decision of the jurors.

The lawyer who has asked you
to appear will decide what testimony is pertinent to the issues and
what information he wishes you to
contribute. This information will
be brought about through what is
called direct examination. Usually
the lawyer in the case has prepared
you prior to your appearance in the
courtroom by giving you examples of
questions that he will ask. In
order for the truth to come out you
must talk together. A court presentation is not necessarily a

spontaneous   presentation.   "You
need to have your thinking together."   For   this   reason   the   lawyer
who requested your testimony will
usually prepare you to describe
tests and test procedures used, and
in general, ask for your opinion
regarding interpretation and use of
such   information.   When   he   has
finished this direct interrogation
you will be cross-examined by the
other lawyer involved in the case.

Cross-examination   gives   the
opposing party an opportunity to
test the evidence given on direct
examination.   The   expert   witness
should be prepared to defend as
objectively as possible any statement he has made upon direct examination.   The   cross-examiner   has
wider latitude in framing questions
and   can   use   leading   questions
concerning any information that has
been given upon direct examination.
He is also permitted hypothetical
questions, and ordinarily he will
attempt to test your knowledge in
your field or ask questions about
other testimony in the case.   If
you can remain alert and listen
carefully to what is asked of you
the cross-examination need not be a
difficult procedure.   If you remember to give your testimony in a
straight forward manner and can
objectively substantiate what you
have said you will have little
difficulty.   If a question is not
understood simply ask the lawyer to
repeat or report that you do not
understand or do not know the
answer. Because the cross-examiner
can ask leading questions about

other testimony in the case it is
well to be aware of exactly what is
within your realm of expertise and
what is not. For example, if you
are asked "Is this child brain-
damaged?" it would be most unwise
for a speech pathologist or audiologist to answer this question because the diagnosis of minimal
brain disfunction or minimal brain
injury is a medical one. The
answer to this question should be
something like, "This is not within
my realm or that's a medical question or I can only evaluate his
behavior."

If you can maintain an attitude of objectivity and not become
emotionally involved, argumenta-
tive, or frightened you can remember this procedure is not a contest
as far as you are concerned. You
are there to give evidence which
will help the court to decide the
issues. It is not the prerogative
of the speech pathologist to "take
sides." Your duty is not to decide
who is right or who is wrong. The
court makes that decision. You
must only give evidence within the
realm of your special knowledge.
Let me demonstrate this with a
hypothetical example. A young man,
with cerebral palsy of the ataxic
type, was being treated for his
speech and voice problem. In
general, his speech rhythm was slow
and distortions of vowels and
consonants were considerable. The
voice quality was breathy and vocal
control was intermittent. The
client, a young college student,
was able to drive from his home to

the office of the speech pathologist as well as into other areas of
the small town in which he lived.
One afternoon he was picked up by a
state trooper on the charge of
drunkenness. When he arrived at
the police station he was allowed
to make the usual phone call and
called the office of the speech
pathologist to inform him that he
was in jail and that the police
wanted to give him the ballon test,
(a test often given in the case of
suspected intoxication). The
client had called to ask the speech
pathologist whether or not he
should allow the police to give him
this test. The speech pathologist
said to himself "I know this boy
isn't drunk. The police are mis-
taken and they are judging his
difficulty in coordination as being
intoxication." Therefore, he advised the client to allow the
police to make whatever tests they
wished. Now, if you were involved
in this case, ask yourself, "What
training do I have to make this
kind of decision for a client?"
Obviously, unless you are a lawyer
you do not have adequate training
to provide the answer for this kind
of legal question because this
question is not within the realm of
the specialty of the speech pathologist. The speech pathologist
should have advised the client to
contact his lawyer or should have
contacted the client's lawyer for
him. This would have been a service the speech pathologist could
have performed within his realm.
Sometimes the individual in the
services of speech pathology and

audiology makes decisions for which he is unprepared and then is unaware of having intruded in a realm that is beyond his knowledge. Essentially, under cross-examination, it is best not to give opinions or make statements concerning questions you have no evidence to substantiate.

In cases of personal injury, the questions revolve around the need to determine preinjury state, the extent of the injury, the prognosis, and finally who is responsible. Here again, the speech pathologist may determine the first three, but the court determines the final question.

An example may illustrate this point. A two-year-old child was in an automobile accident. The mother and child were both injured when a delivery truck for a local department store crashed into their automobile broadside. The child suffered a blow to the right side of the head, concussion, broken ear drum, and lacerations. Speech and language testing was performed by the speech pathologist when the child was 2½ years old and again at 3 years. The question was the extent of damage the child suffered as a result of the accident. Would he need special education or was he functioning in relatively the same category as he had prior to injury? Without preinjury testing the speech pathologist could only relate testing to accepted age norms. In this case, the child was functioning at below age level, and the prognosis was that he would continue to function below age level. The court determined that the truck driver was at fault and the department store was responsible, and the child was awarded a sum of money. Here, the speech pathologist was placed in the position of an expert witness.

Legal involvement may also be as a consultant called by the court to provide information on a patient. Family courts may handle custody cases and need to place a child with the parent best able to provide help. As an example, the court asked the speech pathologist to see a child who was originally being seen by a court social worker who could not understand the child's speech. The judge had a medical report indicating that the child was "normal"; however, at the insistence of the social worker, the speech pathologist was called to evaluate the child for the court. As a result of the evaluation, the mother admitted she had taken another child to the physician in place of the patient. Subsequently, the child was placed with the father and step-mother, and treatment was ordered by the court. In this instance, the speech patholo-gist was a consultant and did not appear in court. In such cases, the remarks, conclu-sions, and opinions of the clinician need not be available to the opposing attorney.

The question of personal ethics and their relationship to professional behavior remains, for the most part, a question that will probably eventually be answered in court. At present psychologists are dealing with the question of unethical sexual in-volvement with patients, but this has not become a serious question for speech patho-logists and audiologists. However, other questions appear as more and more profes-sionals enter private practice. If a practi-tioner works for an agency, hospital, or another practitioner, may he take patients he is treating with him when he opens his own practice? What methods are "ethical" for announcing a new office to patients presently under treatment? Certainly, our professional code of ethics does not provide specific answers to such pressing issues, so issues

must be related to a committee for guidelines. With regard to previous patient
contact, medical protocol usually limits the
practitioner in terms of time (2 years) and
distance (50 miles). What is the responsibility of a practitioner called as a consultant, both to the patient and to the referring practitioner? Does the consultant reveal
his information to both the patient and the
practitioner or only to one? If so, which
one? What is one practitioner's responsibility to another?

For example, one speech pathologist
referred a patient to another for consultation. The second practitioner suspected the
presence of a dangerous vocal disease.
Should the patient be told of this suspicion,
should this be reported to the referring
speech pathologist, or should the patient be
told to get another medical opinion? Improper handling of such a case can lead to a
malpractice suit.

Malpractice suits against speech pathologists are rare at this time, so our guidelines come from other professions. Several
suggestions for avoiding lawsuits may be
appropriate. The plaintiff has the burden of
proving the treatment given was not "standard." The expertise of the provider must be
specified, and appropriate referral should be
made if necessary skills are not present.
Patients have a right to know what procedures
are being suggested, and they also have the
right to refuse treatment, even though this
may be unwise. Always having written consent
from patients or guardians before sending
records to anyone, and keeping records that
are adequate, up-to-date, and as complete as
necessary are deterrents to possible suits.
Each state has its own laws regarding "privileged communication," and knowledge of these
laws may provide guidelines for what can and

should be included in patient records. Above all, adequate malpractice insurance should be kept to cover these possibilities.

   In the role of expert witness or consultant, the speech pathologist is not the major object of the lawsuit; however, in cases of malpractice or libel, he or she is in personal jeopardy. Historically, physicians were only rarely sued for malpractice, but as monetary considerations increased, so did legal suits. The concept of the person against the impersonal corporation, (hospitals and insurance companies) became popular as public awareness increased. Malpractice is covered under the law of torts and includes the concept of negligence; that is, careless conduct which may lead to unintentional harm. Two areas usually are of concern to the speech pathologist. The first is one in which something is placed in or on the patient (tongue blade, palatal lift, mirror, biofeedback apparatus), or touching a patient during treatment. At some point, even doing what one believes is helpful may prove detrimental (moving a patient from wheelchair to bed, or getting a patient to a physician in the midst of a seizure or stroke) as well as hazardous if the patient falls, goes into shock, etc. At present, no lawsuit against a speech pathologist has been reported in legal discussions; however, ASHA's insurance carrier reports three suits pending against audiologists (Carlin, 1977).

   The second area of concern lies in educational testing and placement of a patient with a communication disorder. With the recent passage of legislation mandating appropriate educational placement, professionals making these placements must be accountable for their decisions. Indefensible decisions or improper interpretation of data may be additional areas of attack.

Improper "labeling" may be seen as <u>libelous</u>, while not using appropriate tests for diagnosing problems is considered negligent. The communication specialist who is responsible for the supervision of students may be placed in a compromised position when he becomes responsible for mistakes or misdiagnoses if these would have been avoidable through prudence, forethought, and proper supervision.

All of us should be prepared for the fact that at some time we may have to appear in a court of law as an expert witness or as a participant in a legal suit. Even if we are never called as an expert witness, the preceding suggestions can be helpful in clarifying ambiguous references, unsubstantiated claims, and generalizations in our everyday reporting of case evaluations and therapeutic procedures. If we can manage to take the attitude that we must "stand up in court and prove it," we may take a second look at the evidence we present to justify our claims, whatever they may be.

There is no single road to the truth, nor is truth the certain outcome of scholarship. But men must seek it and--believing to have found a fragment of it--present it to other men for judgment (Officers Committees, 1959)

ACKNOWLEDGMENT

The author wishes to express gratitude to the firm of Funderburk, Murray, Ramsey and Associates, Houston, Texas, for their legal advice.

REFERENCES

Carlin   M: Malpractice   risks   in   speech
pathology and audiology.   Unpublished data

Campbell   CP: Prevent against malpractice
suits.   Washington   State   Psychological
Association Newsletter, Sept. 1975

Glueck S: Law and Psychiatry.   Baltimore,
The Johns Hopkins Press, 1962, p. 181

Liebensen HA, Wepman JM: The Psychologist as
a Witness.   Mundelein,   Illinois,   Callaghon
and Company, 1964, p. 288

Officers   Committees,   1958-59:   Section   of
Insurance, Negligence, and Compensation Law.
1959, p. 198

Overholser W: The Psychiatrist and the Law.
New York, Harcourt, Brace, and Company, 1953,
p. 232

Rada RT, Porch B, Kellner R: Aphasia and the
expert medical witness.   American Academy of
Psychiatry and the Law Bulletin 3(4):   231-
237, 1975

PART II

CHAPTER V

THE CLINICAL ASPECTS OF SPEECH
AND
LANGUAGE PATHOLOGY

Donna R. Fox, Ph.D and R. Ray Battin, Ph.D.

The intent of this chapter is not to
review traditional clinical materials and
procedures in the field, but rather to focus
the attention of the reader on those factors
that are pertinent to private practice: The
clinician in a private setting must make the
best possible use of time available. He must
make the most accurate diagnosis with the
fewest possible samples of behavior.

Scheduling of patients for the speech
pathologist and audiologist may vary significantly. The audiologist schedules by test,
i.e., so much time for air conduction, bone
conduction, SRT, PBM, impedance testing,
hearing aid evaluation, etc. Generally, some
idea of the extent of the patient's problem
is known in advance, and the patient is
allotted time accordingly. If additional
tests are required, they are scheduled at a
later time. The bulk of the audiologist's
work is evaluation, and most patients are
seen on a one-time basis. If the audiologist
sees patients for hearing aid evaluation they
will have several contacts; however, less
time will be spent on subsequent visits than
on the initial one. Standing appointments
for lip reading instruction or auditory
training can be scheduled in the late afternoon. The audiologist must have a strong
referral base for his practice, generally
from physicians specializing in otolaryngology, with general practitioners, pediatri-

cians, and neurologists also a potential referral source, if they are acquainted with the service.

The speech pathologist rarely builds a practice on diagnostic testing alone. On-going treatment makes up the majority of patient contact time. Scheduling must, therefore, provide time for both ongoing treatment and evaluation. As his practice grows, the speech pathologist may schedule all or most of the time with patients in treatment, thus assuring himself of regular income. This can, however, be self-limiting in that referral sources dry up if they are unable to get their patients evaluated when they wish; when this happens, there are no replacements as treatment patients improve. On the other hand, if large blocks of time are left open for evaluations, where do the individuals get treatment? Further, when an evaluation scheduled for a large block of time cancels, the practitioner is punished economically.

The type of practice, age of clients, and ratio of ongoing treatment to evaluation will dictate how a schedule is set up. Generally, school-age children will need to be scheduled for treatment after school hours, with evaluation time early in the day. Adults need to be scheduled over lunch hours or before and after working hours. Again, evaluations can be scheduled during the day, since most adults are willing to take off from work for a single appointment. Those patients not bound by a school or work sched-ule can be placed on the schedule during non-critical times.

While running late on appointments is never advisable, an audiologist can more easily afford running over allotted time for an individual appointment since he can make it up on later patient time or run into the lunch hour or evening hours. However, the speech pathologist cannot afford to repeatedly offend patients with standing appointments. When individuals are seen on a regular basis, they are expected to arrive on time, or else their appointments are shortened accordingly. Otherwise, appointments run late throughout the morning or afternoon. Likewise, it is courteous for the speech pathologist to honor the patient's appointment time, realizing that his other activities are scheduled around this time.

The practitioner who repeatedly is late in seeing ongoing patients soon loses credibility. An organized, systematic approach, which does not take advantage of the patient, allows for the good patient-clinician relationship so critical in achieving treatment goals. Confidence in the clinician's expertise leads to more rapid improvement. This confidence is built not only from the clinical or therapeutic approach, but also from the efficiency and organization of the practice.

Scheduling Evaluations

One of the most difficult scheduling problems is determining just how much time should be allotted for an evaluation so that adequate time is available to assess the problem thoroughly without over-testing, or allowing too much time. Since time is charged for, it must be appropriately utilized.

The preinterview questionnaire for obtaining the patient history information (Appendix) can either be brought to the office at the time of the appointment or mailed in advance, thus facilitating economical use of patient contact time. Experience has shown that wherever possible it is advisable to have the questionnaire, together with a deposit, mailed in advance of the appointment. When a deposit is required, the appointment is generally kept, or if the individual is not able to keep the appointment he will cancel in sufficient time for the time slot to be filled. Receipt of the questionnaire in advance of the evaluation permits the secretary to set up the chart and the speech apthologist to review the material, make notes, and estimate the required evaluation time more accurately. Paper/pencil tests may be administered by the secretary-receptionist, with only direct patient interaction time scheduled with the practitioner. In this way, patients can overlap. Charges for tests vs. those for time with the practitioner must be explained to the patient to avoid criticism, e.g., for only seeing the speech pathologist for 45 minutes. Charges for secretary-administered items must be minimal. It is better to quote an evaluation fee rather than a fee based on time for the intial visit. This gives the examiner more flexibility in choosing tests, interviewing, and counseling with the patient.

Individual speech pathologists will develop their own diagnostic battery of tests. The following examples of scheduling are presented as a guide for the beginning practitioner:

Stuttering--Adult. Generally an hour can be scheduled for the adult stutterer, if the preinterview questionnaire has been received in advance and if the speech pathologist has a good secretary who can prepare the chart properly and monitor paper/pencil tests such as the Iowa attitude toward stuttering test, the Rotter or MMPI, or whatever instruments the speech pathologist is qualified to give and interpret.

Stuttering--Child. One to two hours of direct contact is the usual time needed depending upon whether the examiner believes that intelligence testing should be a part of the evaluation battery and is qualified to give such tests. Parent counseling may take a major portion of the time allotment if the child is a pre-schooler.

Articulation Disorders. The preinterview questionnaire will provide the examiner with good insight into what is required in the way of testing. Previous testing will be listed and should be forwarded prior to the appointment. However, on occasion, the parent will play "see if you can find out what I know about my child" and does not list other agency contacts. A method of eliciting both running or conversational speech and a language sample can utilize the same time frame and probably should be tape recorded for reference and further study if necessary. Approximately 1-1½ hours is usual for this type of disorder. Time allotted may also depend on whether or not the practitioner uses a screening device or refers to a consultant for estimating intellectual function.

Craniofacial Abnormalities. In this category of disorders, the speech pathologist will generally need to know the specific questions of the referral agency or physician. In the case of adults, the questions may revolve around vocational placement, while with children the questions are often related to surgical intervention regarding structural ade-quacy. If the question is one of velo-

pharyngeal competency, and extensive
medical, dental, social, and psychologic
studies have already been accomplished,
then the time for articulatory and
resonance testing may be minimal. However, if the speech and language assessment is the entry point for study, then
much more time for testing and counseling may need to be allotted.

Voice. Individuals with voice problems
generally can be evaluated in about 45
minutes to one hour, depending on whether a medical status report on the larynx
is available prior to scheduling. For
example, initial contact with a laryn-
gectomy patient may be 10-15 minutes in
some cases to one hour in others, depending on the prior knowledge of the
patient and his problem. A child with
nodules on the vocal cords may be tested
in 30 minutes, while a professional
voice user may require one hour and 15
minutes. All of these considerations
depend upon the skill and adeptness of
the practitioner; as with all learned
skills, practice in testing and listening must be continuous.

Aphasia. There are numerous, strong test
instruments for aphasia. Most take an
hour or more to administer with interpretation providing comparable information. The aphasiologist will tend to
use the instrument that provides him
with the most useful information for
establishing a treatment program. Care
must be taken to not be test-bound, for
frequently a screening instrument
coupled with acute observation skills
will provide the examiner with the
needed information without costing the
patient in time and fatigue. A screening instrument can be adapted by the

examiner or he can use one of the existing instruments. It should adequately
assess remaining language skills, both
receptive and expressive, and give some
estimate of prognosis. A strong pre-
insult history will be invaluable in
assessing remaining skills and outlining
realistic goals.

Delayed Language. Evaluating the child with
a language delay probably mandates a
team approach. It is necessary to
delineate etiological factors such as
hearing loss, autism, mental retarda-
tion, and childhood schizophrenia. The
speech pathologist's contribution to the
evaluation is the determination of
language functioning as it relates to
the level of overall abilities. The
treatment program may be a joint venture
or may be solely in the hands of the
speech pathologist. Time allotted for
evaluating the language delayed child
will vary significantly. The clinical
and professional training of the speech
pathologist will dictate whether intelligence and audiological assessment is a
part of the test battery.

Summary

Adults often do not require lengthy,
numerous test instruments, since information
can be obtained from their work history. The
child's school history and achievement tests
provide valuable information to the experienced speech pathologist, thus shortening the
testing time without sacrificing critical
information needed for a thorough diagnostic
review.

Realistic times should be allotted for
evaluations, allowing for adequate analysis

of the problem but eliminating unnecessary
testing.   It is   better to reschedule the
patient for additional study than to feel
compelled to fill allotted time.   In this
way, the practitioner minimizes fees to the
patient and maximizes efficient utilization
of patient contact time.

APPENDIX

CHAPTER V

Please return the questionnaire with deposit to:

THE BATTIN CLINIC
Psycholinguistics-Clinical Psychology-Audiology
3931 Essex Lane, Suite F
Houston, Texas 77027

Your evaluation
appointment is:

Day _____

Date _____

Time _____

Pre-Interview Questionnaire
for Children with Speech, Language or Learning Disabilities

Date _____

Name _____ Age _____ Birthdate _____

Address _____ Zip _____ Sex: □ M □ F

_____ Phone _____

Person completing form _____

Relationship to client _____

Name of referring doctor or agency _____

Their specialty _____

Address _____ Phone _____

Has the child had any previous testing either at school or through a private agency? If

so, give the name of the agency and the dates tested:

Name _____ Date _____

Address _____

(Please request that copies of results of all testing be sent to this office)

Why is this testing being requested? (Use back of page if needed)

101

FAMILY INFORMATION

Father's Name _____ Age _____

Address _____

Occupation _____ Business Phone _____

Employer _____

Address _____

Health: ☐ Good   ☐ Fair   ☐ Poor   Education completed _____

Mother's Name _____ Age _____

Address _____ Phone _____

Business Address _____ Business Phone _____

Occupation (state full- or part-time) _____

Health: ☐ Good   ☐ Fair   ☐ Poor   Education completed _____

List all children in the family from the oldest to the youngest:

NAME   AGE   GENERAL HEALTH

102

Do any of the other children have special problems?

Are any of the children adopted?

Others living in the home:

NAME   AGE   RELATIONSHIP TO CHILD
_____

Is any language other than English spoken in the home?

Have there been any changes in the family group (such as death, divorce, frequent change of address, prolonged absence or illness of either parent, etc.)? Describe:

BIRTH HISTORY

Weight of child at birth _____ Was child full term? _____

Were there any unusual factors relating to the pregnancy (such as toxemia, X-ray treatments, RH negative, German measles, other illnesses, drugs or medication)?

Type of birth: ☐ normal ☐ induced ☐ forceps ☐ Caesarean ☐ breech
                ☐ premature

Were there any physical deformities or malformations observed at birth? Describe:

DEVELOPMENTAL HISTORY

In early childhood, did the child have any feeding problems, such as poor control of sucking, food allergies, digestive upsets, etc? ☐ Yes ☐ No
Describe:

Do you feel that the child was late or had difficulty in the development of the following behaviors? □ Yes   □ No

GIVE AGE OF DEVELOPMENT

Sitting _____   Walking _____

Eating solid foods _____   Self-feeding _____

Crawling _____   Self-dressing _____

Standing alone _____   Bladder & bowel control _____

Which hand does the child prefer? _____

Is there a family history of left handedness? _____

Does the child have any present problems in eating, sleeping, bladder control, or with constipation?

(Developmental History continued)

Does he complain of aches, pains, headaches, stomachaches?

Have any of these nervous habits been observed?

	YES	NO		YES	NO
Nail biting	☐	☐	Pulling at hair or clothing	☐	☐
Thumb sucking	☐	☐	Facial tics	☐	☐
Stuttering	☐	☐	Other	☐	☐

Do any of these terms apply to your child?

	YES	NO		YES	NO
Timid	☐	☐	Very stubborn	☐	☐
Easily embarrassed	☐	☐	Bossy	☐	☐
Sensitive to criticism	☐	☐	Irritable	☐	☐
Often fearful	☐	☐	Impudent	☐	☐
Often nervous	☐	☐	Very disorderly	☐	☐
Jealous	☐	☐	Exceptionally quiet	☐	☐
Overly neat and particular	☐	☐	Excitable	☐	☐

At any time in his development, did any of these behaviors occur?

Frequent crying	☐	Destructiveness	☐	
Clinging to mother	☐	Lying	☐	
Much daydreaming	☐	Frequent fighting	☐	
Withdrawal from others	☐	Stealing	☐	
Running from others	☐	Unusual sexual behavior	☐	
Temper tantrums	☐	Other	☐	

Do you believe that your child is now well coordinated in walking, using his hands, running, riding a trike or bike, etc.? ☐ Yes ☐ No

Does he fall frequently? ☐ Yes ☐ No

MEDICAL FACTORS

Present weight _____ Present height _____

Doctor most familiar with problem _____

Doctor's address _____

Date and type of last medical examination _____

(Medical continued)

Childhood diseases:

	YES	NO		YES	NO
Measles	☐	☐	Rheumatic fever	☐	☐
Mumps	☐	☐	Chicken pox	☐	☐
Whooping cough	☐	☐	Pneumonia	☐	☐
Other					

Were there any complications with the above, such as high and persistent fever, convulsions, persistent muscle weakness, etc.?

Is the child subject to frequent colds, frequent sore throats? _____

Has he had allergies, asthma, hayfever, etc. _____

Does he tend to breathe with his mouth open? _____

Has the child had any operations? _____ Specify: _____

Have tonsils and adenoids been removed? _____ When _____

Has he had any trouble with his ears, such as earaches, infections, running ears, evidence of hearing loss? _____

Has hearing been tested? _____ When _____

Has he ever worn glasses or had any difficulty with his eyes? _____

Has he been referred for orthodontia? _____

Has the child had special physical examinations of any kind? Please explain. _____

EDUCATION

Present grade _____ Name of school _____

Address of School _____

Teacher's name _____

Did he attend nursery school? _____ How long? _____

At what age did he attend kindergarten? _____

Does he like school? _____ Does he like his teacher? _____

Are any school subjects difficult for him? _____

Has he ever failed or skipped a grade? _____

(Education continued)

What are his best subjects? _____

Have you discussed his problems with his teacher? _____

Does he attend any special classes? _____
e.g. speech therapy, language development, reading clinic, etc.

How does the teacher describe your child's behavior in school:

☐ poor work habits   ☐ does not pay attention   ☐ does not listen

☐ does not use time and materials effectively   ☐ written work careless

☐ does not discipline himself

Other _____

What kinds of grades does your child receive?

☐ A's   ☐ A's & B's   ☐ B's   ☐ B's & C's   ☐ C's   ☐ C's & D's   ☐ D's

☐ D's & F's   ☐ F's   ☐ Inconsistent grades   Describe: _____

What type of study habits does your child demonstrate at home?

☐ Spends at least an hour a day on homework   ☐ Has a quiet place to study

☐ Able to work with one or both parents   ☐ Appears to know material at home but
                                               not in school

SOCIAL HISTORY

What is your type of residence?

    □ Separate home   □ Apartment   □ Trailer   Other _____

Where does your child usually play? _____

Are there any children his age in the neighborhood? _____

Does he prefer to play alone? _____

Is he a leader or a follower in his play? _____

Does he prefer older or younger children? _____

Does he have a special friend? _____

Does he play well with brothers or sisters? _____

Does his father play with the child frequently? _____

Describe the child's most frequent playmates:

(Social History continued)

How many hours a day does he watch TV _____

What are your most frequent discipline problems with this child?

_____

Who does the disciplining? _____

How do you discipline? _____

What do you consider the child's main social assets?

LANGUAGE DEVELOPMENT

How old was the child when he first started to use words? _____

How old was the child when he first made sentences? _____

Does he have a speech problem? _____ Describe:

When did you first notice it? _____ If no speech

problem now, did he ever have one? _____ Describe:

112

Has the child had any help for this difficulty? _____

DATES _____

Has anyone teased him about his speech or criticized him excessively? _____

How did he react? _____

Do you think his speech has changed in the last six months? _____

What do you believe is the main cause of his speech difficulty? _____

Briefly describe your child's personality (use back of paper)

I give my permission for my child to be tested (both parents must sign).

_____

_____

113

BILLING INFORMATION

Who is responsible for the bill?

Name _____ Phone _____

Address _____

Business Address _____

Business Phone _____ Occupation _____

Insurance forms will be filled out if you provide the form. However, please note that we do not accept assignment and you, NOT THE INSURANCE COMPANY, will be responsible for the charges.

Evaluation fees are payable at the time of the testing unless advance arrangements have been made with this office.

FIGURE 1

CHAPTER VI

REPORT WRITING FOR PRIVATE PRACTITIONERS

Kenneth J. Knepflar, Ph.D.

As specialists in the field of communication disorders, all speech pathologists and
audiologists are confronted with the responsibility of preparing written reports of
various types. While effective reports are
important for professionals in all work
settings, they are of particular significance
for those in private practice. Letters and
reports to those who refer patients and to
those who cooperate in patients' treatment
programs are vital to the ultimate success of
those who expect to build and maintain private practices in speech pathology and/or
audiology. In many instances reports provide
the major basis upon which judgements are
made concerning the diagnostic and clinical
abilities of private practitioners. If a
physician, for example, receives no written
communication from the professional person to
whom he has referred his patient, he is very
likely to search for other, more communicative referral sources. Similarly, if he
receives only a brief thank you note or an
impersonal "checklist" report, with no specific narrative account, he is apt to be skep-
tical concerning the professional capabilities and ethical responsibilities of the
individual speech pathologist or audiologist.

Butler (1976) in her introduction to the
handbook, Report Writing in the Field of
Communication Disorders (Knepflar, 1976),
made this statement concerning the importance
of report writing skills to our profession:

While institutions of higher education may vary to some degree in the
emphasis placed upon diagnostic
reports and the preparation thereof, all clinicians, aborning and
fully-fledged, need to develop a
high level of competency in the
endeavor. Carefully-honed and
highly-polished, the ability to
transmit clinical activities and
judgements will stand you in good
stead all the days of your professional life.

Many texts have been written in psychology,
psychiatry, and other fields to train students and professionals to write reports
(Huber, 1961, Klopfer, 1960; Tallent, 1976).
One report writing text in the field of
communication disorders has appeared
(Knepflar, 1976). Several journal articles
have also been written that are of value to
those speech pathologists and audiologists
who would like to improve their report writing capabilities (English and Lillywhite,
1963; Jerger, 1962; Moore, 1969; Pannbacker,
1975). Sections of a few textbooks in speech
pathology, particularly those in the area of
diagnosis, have published sections having to
do with report writing (Emerick and Hatten,
1974; Johnson, et al., 1961; Nation and Aram,
1977). While the above-mentioned report
writing references may be of assistance to
speech and language pathologists and audiologists, regardless of their work settings,
this chapter is specifically aimed at those
in private practice and those planning to
enter this rapidly growing and highly challenging area of the profession.

In her handbook, Private Practice, Fox
(1971), explains how private practice differs
from other work settings.

In the protected shelter of an institution such as the school, the institution and not the profession is most important. In the hospital, agency or clinic, the organization and not the profession is of primary importance. In private practice, however, the practitioner alone represents his profession. His practice reflects his effectiveness and his sense of responsibility to his patient.

Reports written by private practitioners should reflect a high degree of professionalism, high ethical standards, and legal responsibility. Inaccuracy, vagueness, ambiguity, wordiness, and meaningless professional jargon all reflect on the individual capabilities of the practitioner. For those in private practice, there is no large organization or institution to back up such errors in judgement. The private practitioner must communicate effectively through both oral and written language.

Basic Concepts in Writing Reports

Obviously, the major objective of any report must be to communicate specific diagnostic and/or clinical findings about a patient. A second objective is to teach the reader something about the field of speech and language disorders. A third objective is to assist in building authentic meaningful relationships with other professionals.

If private practitioners in the field of communication disorders are to be successful in accomplishing these objectives, they must consider a basic fact of professional life. Private practitioners spend most of their working hours seeing patients. Therefore,

much of their report writing is done during
evenings and what would otherwise be free
time. It is particularly important, therefore, that a system of report writing be
developed, whereby reports are concise,
complete, well organized, and, above all,
honest.

Conciseness

Many training programs in speech pathology and audiology encourage students to
write lengthy reports that may run seven or
eight typewritten pages. Very few private
practitioners have time to write such detailed reports. Furthermore, most of the
referring physicians do not have time to read
them. Effective reports present the essential facts without lengthy illustrations,
quotations, and insignificant details.
Superfluous adjectives and adverbs and literary embellishments should be eliminated.

Completeness

To combine conciseness with completeness
is a difficult task, but not an impossible
one. Many lengthy reports fail to include
all essential ingredients. For example, they
may not mention results of hearing tests as
part of an articulation or voice evaluation,
while including lists of childhood diseases
that have no etiological significance to the
problem being evaluated.

Organization

If sections of a report are not properly
labeled (i.e., background information, articulation, voice, language, etc.), readers
often have difficulty locating information

and separating pieces of unrelated information. If, however, a basic preprinted organizational outline is followed during the testing and interviewing processes, all pieces of information regarding a specific topic are together and can be easily organized into a meaningful, well-structured report.

It is not the purpose of this chapter to suggest a specific organization structure for diagnostic or clinical reports. Many acceptable outlines for reports have been recommended. We must organize our reports in a manner with which we can be comfortable. Further information regarding the organization of diagnostic reports appears later in this chapter.

Honesty

In the report writing handbook this statement was made (Knepflar, 1976):

> It is of great importance for each of us, not only in report writing, but in all of our professional activities, to be honest about what we know and what we do not know. A competent speech pathologist should not behave like a frustrated neurologist, laryngologist, or psychiatrist. An audiologist must not behave like a frustrated otologist. Reports must convey our findings, but we must be willing to admit that we do not have all of the answers (p.6).

It is vital that reports present facts and that all subjective information, such as clinical impressions, be properly labeled. Conclusions should never be stated that cannot be properly backed up by the evaluation findings. If speech and language pathologists in private practice make statements they cannot substantiate, they are likely to lose the respect of the colleagues upon whom they depend for referrals. It is also important to keep in mind the possibility of legal problems if unsupported statements are made (see Fox, this volume).

Specialized Reports

Most private practitioners in the field of communication disorders find it necessary to familiarize themselves with many kinds of reporting and record keeping that were not included in their academic training. For example, in addition to their diagnostic and clinical work in their offices, many private practitioners find themselves performing evaluative and treatment services in hospitals, convalescent hospitals, rehabilitation centers, and in the homes of patients (often through contractual agreements with home health agencies). Most such facilities require detailed treatment plans, daily progress notes, and periodic summary reports in addition to the original evaluative or diagnostic report (see Barr, this volume).

Diagnostic Reports

Ordinarily, the most challenging report writing responsibility of speech-language pathologists or audiologists is the complete report of the initial evaluation of patients. It is in this report that tests must be summarized and interpreted. It is also in the diagnostic report that specialists in the field of communication disorders must provide a specific, clear explanation of every aspect of the patient's communicative functioning. Diagnostic reports provide the foundation for all future treatment plans, summary reports, and progress notes. Many organizational formats for diagnostic reports have been proposed (Emerick and Hatten, 1974; Johnson et al., 1961; Knepflar, 1976; Nation and Aram, 1977; Sanders, 1972). Regardless of the specific content outline that may be selected, it is vital that reports contain all available information presented in an organized, readable manner. This is particularly important for private practitioners, whose professional reputations in the medical community in which they practice often rest heavily on their ability to convey diagnostic information to other professionals who are cooperating in the treatment of a patient.

A major weakness of many diagnostic reports written by speech-language pathologists is that they cover only limited, isolated information regarding the patient's major problem, with no mention of the status of other aspects of communicative functioning. For example, if a child has an articulation disorder, the report may be limited to statements regarding articulation development, articulation tests, and recommendations for an articulation treatment program. Such a report, with no mention of language, voice, or speech fluency is incomplete. Even if no specific testing was done in some areas of communicative functioning, clinical statements should be made concerning each of these areas. For a more complete statement of this philosophy see Chapter III of the report writing handbook (Knepflar, 1976).

The Report Letter

Some speech-language pathologists and audiologists, particularly those in private practice, select a personal letter to the referral source in lieu of a more formally

structured report. The report-letter is
particularly appropriate when the major
purpose is to acknowledge a referral, to
exlain initial impressions after a first
interview, or to explain that a more complete
diagnostic report will follow after further
testing has been completed.

A relatively brief letter is often sent
to a child's classroom teacher, together with
copies of printed information concerning how
to assist that particular child in the classroom. When complete diagnostic information
is to be communicated, a well-organized
report should be sent rather than a lengthy,
rambling letter.

When the more complete report format is
used, it should always be accompanied by a
brief cover letter to the referring physician, in which there is an opportunity to
express thanks for making the referral.
Copies of the report, with appropriate cover
letters, should be sent to other professionals who are cooperating in the patient's
treatment. This not only improves communication among members of the medical team, but
also provides an effective, ethical avenue
for effective public relations.

Insurance Reports

Most private practitioners earn a significant portion of their incomes through
payments from private insurance companies and
federally sponsored (Medicare) or state
sponsored (Medicaid, worker's compensation,
and state disability) health insurance plans.
Each insurance company has its specific forms
that must be correctly completed by the
patient and by the health services provider.
Each insurance policy describes the specific
benefits that are covered. Some descriptions

of benefits for speech pathology services are vague and confusing. If payments are to be expected, reports must be accurate and written in clear language that can be understood by the individuals responsible for accepting or rejecting claims. It is particularly important that diagnostic statements be complete and specific. Most insurance forms have been designed for use by physicians and do not lend themselves to use by speech-language pathologists and audiologists. To enhance the chances of acceptance by insurance companies, the prepared form usually should be accompanied by a summary report and a letter from the referring physician. This letter should state specific medical diagnosis and a recommendation that speech-language pathology treatment services be initiated. In many instances it is advisable that the physician's letter mention the number of sessions recommended per week.

Many insurance claims are initially rejected by insurance companies. Such denials should not be considered final. Frequently such decisions are made by individuals who are unfamiliar with the terminology of speech-language pathology and audiology. If, after reading the provisions of the patient's insurance policy, the private practitioner believes that communication disorder services should be covered, the decision should be appealed. Such appeals should be accompanied by additional letters of explanation from the speech-language pathologist and/or the referring physician. Letters and telephone calls from the patient and/or his family can also be of assistance in reversing decisions regarding insurance eligibility.

Progress Notes

As part of their training, most specialists in the field of communication disorders
have been instructed to keep daily progress
notes. Many people, after a number of years
of professional experience, however, fail to
keep such session-by-session records of their
clinical work. Others write abbreviated,
incomplete notes that may be meaningful to
them, but would be of little value to anyone
else who might need to review them at a later
date. For private practitioners, much of
whose clinical work is paid for through
private and government health insurance
programs, daily progress notes are not only
desirable but, in many instances, essential.
In some cases, payment has been denied because progress notes have not been available,
or because the progress notes did not provide
evidence that the clinical techniques were
compatible with the original diagnosis and
treatment plan. In other instances, progress
notes have been so general and so sketchy,
that a new clinician taking over the responsibility of treating a patient finds them of
little or no value.

The following statement regarding requirements for good progress notes was suggested in the handbook, Report Writing in the
Field of Communication Disorders (Knepflar,
1976, p. 23):

Good progress notes will usually include
the following:

(1) Brief notes concerning specific
     clinical management techniques and
     materials used.
(2) Interpretation of how the patient
     responded, and statements regarding
     the patient's progress.

(3)   Suggestions or assignments given to
       the patient and, when appropriate,
       recommendations for the next ses-
       sion.

Summary Reports

Some private insurance companies and
most federal, state, and local medical insurance plans (Medicare, Medicaid, worker's
compensation, and state or local crippled
children's services) require periodic summary
reports before a continuation of treatment
can be authorized. Such summary reports,
even when not required by an outside agency,
should be prepared periodically by private
practitioners in order to assure continued
communication with referring physicians and
cooperating specialists in other fields. A
final summary report at the time treatment is
terminated is of particular importance. In
some instances, requests for such reports
will be received years after treatment has
been completed. Without clearly stated
progress notes and summary reports, it is
difficult, if not impossible, to fulfill such
requests.

Summary reports should always include
information concerning the specific clinical
approaches that were beneficial in treating a
patient, those that were not helpful, or
those that were resisted by a patient.
Statements of test scores, without a narrative presentation of clincial data, are of
little value to individuals who need to
continue a patient's treatment at a later
date.

The Writing Process

Many individuals who are very adept at communicating orally have feelings of insecurity regarding their technical writing abilities. It is impossible in this chapter to present a short course on the development of writing skills. It is possible, however, to refer current and future private practitioners to many available sources that can aid in breaking down barriers to effective report writing.

A number of excellent report writing texts have been written that can be used as references for those who wish to refine their writing skills. Jones (1971) is a particularly useful source for those who feel insecure regarding word choice, grammar, and syntax in scientific writing.

Another text on writing style (Strunk and White, 1959) presents the following advice to beginning writers, which is especially valid for those in private practice:

> The beginner should. . .begin by turning resolutely away from all devices that are popularly believed to indicate style--all mannerisms, tricks, adornments. The approach to style is by way of plainness, simplicity, orderliness, sincerity . . . the first piece of advice is this: to achieve style, begin by affecting none--that is, place yourself in the background. A careful and honest writer does not need to worry about style.

Texts on report writing in psychology and psychiatry often have been used by specialists in the field of communication disorders. Most notable among them are Huber, 1961; Klopfer, 1960; and Tallent, 1976.

Among these texts, Huber is particularly helpful. In Chapter VI, "How to Put it in Writing," he points out that reports should not be subtle, and that report writing should not take on a fiction style. He says:

> Words for their own sake are inappropriate in clinical reports. Even more important: the reader should not be "left on his own;" there should be no place for him to "read into" the report. He should be informed explicitly; he should know exactly what the reporter means. The statements in a report are apt to influence the reader greatly in making important decisions about a patient's life. These statements should therefore be clear and unequivocal (p.71).

In Chapter V of the handbook, <u>Report Writing in the Field of Communication Disorders</u> (Knepflar, 1976), the following twelve basic rules for writing style are explained, with frequent quotations from actual clinical reports:

1. Use specific language. Avoid ambiguous terms.

2. Use nontechnical language that can be understood by the reader. Define terms that may not be universally comprehended. Avoid jargon.

3. Use complete words which may be clearly understood by readers. Avoid abbreviations.

4.   Use a variety of language styles
        and word selections, according
        to the needs of the report.
        Avoid stereotypy.

5.   Use specific, accurate, brief
        sentences. Avoid verbosity and
        needless words.

6.   Convey a sincere, serious pro-
        fessional attitude in your
        writing. Avoid flippancy.

7.   Use complete verb forms and
        correct punctuation. Avoid
        contractions and hyphens.

8.   Use positive statements that
        show what testing or observa-
        tions have revealed. Avoid
        qualifiers and noncommittal
        language.

9.   Use personal pronouns when they
        are the natural way to make a
        clear statement. Avoid awkward
        circumlocutions.

10.   Use accurate, descriptive lan-
        guage that can be supported by
        fact. Avoid exaggeration and
        overstatement.

11.   Select the exact words you need
        to express a specific concept or
        idea. Avoid misusing words.

12.   Use active-verb construction
        whenever possible. Avoid pas-
        sive-verb forms (pp. 29-42).

    In addition to the dictionary, Roget's
Thesarus, and other commonly used word references, a number of books are currently avail-

able to assist speakers and writers in improving their ability to use the language with
more ease and accuracy. Among the most
helpful to private practitioners in the
fields of speech-language pathology and audiology are: Harper Dictionary of Contemporary
Usage (Morris and Morris, 1975); Dictionary
of Problem Words and Expressions (Shaw,
1975); Sisson's Word and Expression Locater
(Sisson, 1975); and Words Into Type
(Skillen, Gay, et al., 1974).

Semantic Aspects of Report Writing

One of the objectives of reports, as was
stated earlier in this chapter, is to educate
the reader concerning the field of communication disorders. Few physicians, dentists,
and other specialists who refer patients to
speech-language pathologists and audiologists
are well-informed about our profession.
Often reports written by speech and language
specialists fail to accomplish the objective
of teaching the reader, merely because of the
unfortunate choice of words carrying negative
or confusing labels that can be easily misinterpreted.

The speech-language pathologist in
private practice is expected to know what he
is talking and writing about. A technical
and/or scientific word that is used incor-
rectly or in a manner that can be easily
misinterpreted may have a negative influence
on a private practitioner's professional
reputation. Similarly, such unfortunate
semantic errors can prevent readers from
improving their understanding of the field of
communication disorders. For example, many
report writers use terms such as, "I feel
that," "It is my impression that," and "It is
probable that," so frequently that the reader
gets the overall impression that the report

contains few, if any, facts or that the
writer is afraid to commit himself and make
definite factual statements without protec-
tive qualifiers. If you are not reasonably
convinced that a statement is true, perhaps
it should be deleted from the report, or at
least reserved for the "Clinical Impressions"
section of the report.

The language of the field of communication disorders is laden with technical terms
that mean little or nothing to many of the
people for whom reports are written. If
technical terminology is used, it should be
defined. If scientific jargon can be eliminated entirely and clear descriptive language
used in its place, the readability of the
report will be improved.

Additional information regarding the
semantic aspects of report writing for
speech-language pathologists and audiologists
can be found in Chapter VI of the report
writing handbook (Knepflar, 1976).

For those who are just embarking on the
private practice adventure and who feel the
need to familiarize themselves with reports
of various kinds, many exemplary reports
appear in the appendices of texts by Knepflar
(1976) and Nation and Aram (1977).

Final Considerations in Report Writing

Many diagnostic and clinical reports
have been prepared which would have been a
source of embarrassment if they had not been
carefully corrected, edited, and, in some
instances, rewritten before they were sent.
Reports have been signed, sealed, and delivered, containing arbitrary or vague statements, awkard language, unsubstantiated
conclusions, insignificant, superfluous de-

tails, glaring omissions of vital information, incorrect test scores, and obvious
typographical errors. Private practitioners
cannot afford to be represented by these
kinds of substandard reports. If rough
drafts of reports are written in longhand or
typed by the speech-language pathologist or
audiologist, they should be read again and
again before being submitted for final typing. If they are dictated to a secretary or
into a dictation machine, they should be
typed in rough draft form and edited before a
final typing. The final draft should always
be proofread before a signature is affixed.
Errors made and overlooked one day can often
be identified and corrected the next day.

Those who know they do not write well
must not resort to brief check-list reports,
short notes, or telephone calls to their
referral sources if they expect to build,
maintain, and expand their private practices.
Our patients do not get over their speech and
language disorders if they do not speak, we
do not get over our writing problems if we do
not write! Writing courses are available in
colleges, universities, and through community
adult education programs. We all have
friends, colleagues, family members, or
employees who can read our reports and give
helpful suggestions. We should read the
rough drafts of our reports as we would those
of a student if we were teaching. We should
read our own reports as if we were the recip-
ients. A report that is appropriate for a
physician might be totally inappropriate for
a classroom teacher. We are specialists in
the field of communication disorders. We
must communicate!

If this chapter and its list of references is of benefit to readers in helping to
solve their "disorders of written communication," one objective of the chapter will have

been accomplished.   If those entering private
practice   realize   more   vividly   the   vital
importance that report writing may have in
their professional futures, a second objective will have been satisfied.

REFERENCES

Bangs T, Rister A: Efficiency in report writing. Hrg and Sp News 37: 12-16, 1969

Butler K: Introduction, in Knepflar, K. J.: Report writing in the Field of Communication Disorders, Danville, Ill., Interstate, 1976, p IX-X

Darley FL: Diagnosis and Appraisal of Communication Disorders, Englewood Cliffs, N. J., Prentice-Hall, 1964, 152 pp

Emerick LL, Hatten JT: Diagnosis and Evaluation in Speech Pathology, Englewood Cliffs, N. J., Prentice-Hall, 1974, 333 pp

English RE, Lillywhite HS: A semantic approach to clinical reporting in speech pathology. Asha, 5: 647-650, 1963

Fox DR: (ed) Private Practice, Guidelines for Speech Pathology and Audiology, Danville, Ill., Interstate, 1971, p. 3

Good R: The written language of rehabilitation medicine: meaning and usages. Arch Phys Med and Rehab 15: 29-36, 1970

Hammond KR, Allen JM, Jr.: Writing Clinical Reports, Englewood Cliffs, N.J., Prentice-Hall, 1953, 235 pp

Huber JT: Report Writing in Psychology and Psychiatry. New York, Harper and Row, 1961, p 111

Jerger J: Scientific writing can be reasonable. Asha 4: 191-104, 1962

Johnson W, Darley FL, Spriestersbach D: Diagnostic Methods in Speech Pathology. New York, Harper and Row, 1963, 347 pp

Jones WP: Writing Scientific Papers and Reports (ed 6). Dubuque, Iowa, Wm. C. Brown Co. 1971, 361 pp

Klopfler WG: The Psychological Report. New York, Grune and Stratton, 1960, 146 pp

Knepflar KJ: Is full time private practice for you? Calif. J. Comm. Dis. 2: 143-146, 1972

Knepflar KJ: The private practitioner's accountability under ASHA's code of ethics. Unpublished paper presented at ASHA convention, Detroit, Mich. 10/12/73

Knepflar KJ: Report Writing in the Field of Communication Disorders. Danville, Ill., Interstate, 1976, 100 pp

Laguaite J, Riviere M, Fuller C: Problems of terminology, ASHA 7: 152-155, 1965

Mayman M: Style focus, language and content of an ideal psychologic test report, J. Proj. Tech. 23: 453, 1959

Merrill PW: The principles of poor writing, Sci. Mon. 64: 72-74, 1947

Moore MV: Pathological writing, ASHA, 11: 535-38, 1969

Morris W, Morris M: Harper Dictionary of Contemporary Usage, New York, Harper and Row, 1975, 648 pp

Nation JE, Aram DM: Diagnosis of Speech and Language Disorders, St. Louis, C.V. Mosby, Co., 1977

Pannbacker, M.: Diagnostic report writing. J of Sp and Hrg Dis 40: 367-379, 1975.

Sanders LJ: Procedure Guides for Evaluation of Speech and Language Disorders in Children (ed. 3).   Danville, Ill., Interstate, 1972, 131 pp

Shaw H: Dictionary of Problem Words and Expressions, New York, McGraw-Hill, 1975, 262 pp

Sisson AF: Sisson's word and expression locater, West Nyack, New York, Parker, 1975, 371 pp

Skillen ME, Gay RM: Words into Type (ed. 3). Englewood Cliffs, N.J., Prentice-Hall, 1974, 583 pp

Strunk W, Jr., White EB: The Elements of Style.   New York, MacMillan, 1959, 71 pp

Tallent N: On individualizing the psychologist's clinical evaluation, J Clin Psy 14: 243-245, 1958

Tallent N: Psychological Report Writing, Englewood Cliffs, N.J., Prentice-Hall, 1976, 262 pp

Woodford FP: Sounder thinking through clear writing, Sci. 156: 743-744, 1967

CHAPTER VII

SPEECH PATHOLOGY SERVICES IN HOME CARE AGENCIES

Nona Lee Barr, M.A.

Introduction

Home health agencies provide an opportunity for speech pathologists to see certain
communicatively impaired patients, and at the
same time provide work settings for private
practitioners. "Coordinated home care" has
been defined as a program "that is centrally
administered and that, through coordinated
planning, evaluation, and follow-up procedures for physician-directed medical, nursing, social, and rehabilitation provides
services to selected patients at home"
(Cowdry and Steinberg, 1971).

Coordinated home care gives more to the
patient than just the physician's care in his
own home. It provides him with health services that are usually confined to institutional settings--services that he would have
to forego were they not delivered to his home
by a centrally administered agency. To the
physician, home care is of invaluable assistance, permitting him to give comprehensive
care of high quality to his homebound patient, with a minimum expenditure of time and
energy on his part. Nurses, physical therapists, social workers, speech pathologists,
and other professional workers upon whose
help he has come to rely in his hospital work
are available to him to care for the homebound patient. In addition, home care re-
duces the length of hospital stay and pre-
vents or delays the commitment of many chron-

ically ill and physically disabled patients
to custodial institutions.

The first home care program in this
country was initiated by the Boston Dispensary in 1796 so that the sick poor might be
cared for at less expense to the community,
children would not be deprived of the loving
care of their parents, the offspring of the
elderly and disabled might express gratitude
and tenderness to their parents which is
their due, and charity would be more refined
and more secret (Cowdry and Steinberg).

The Boston Dispensary program was inau-
gurated at a time when the home was the preferred locale for care of the sick and when
hospitals were reserved for the poor who
could not afford the luxury of sick care in
their homes. The program was designed to
relieve the poor of the need for demeaning
hospitalizations and commitment to poor
houses (Cowdry and Steinberg, 1971).

With the advent of scientific medicine,
medical care shifted to the hospitals, in
which skilled personnel and complex and
costly equipment for diagnosis and effective
medical and surgical treatment were readily
available. However, after World War II, the
number of hospital beds in many communities
began to fall short of the need. Demand for
skilled personnel began to exceed the supply,
and hospital costs rose and continued to rise
precipitously over the general cost-of-living
increase. Obviously, that precious and
expensive hospital care should be reserved
for those in true medical need, and many
chronically ill patients could be managed
well at home, provided the necessary services
could be brought to them.

The growth of home care as a major mode
of health care delivery was given impetus by

the implementation of Medicare. Before 1966, the United States Public Health Service could identify only 70 programs of coordinated home care. By January 1969, 2,194 home health agencies were certified for participation in the Medicare program.

The National League for Nursing in 1975 listed in the Directory of Home Health Agencies 2,247 certified to participate in the Medicare program (Cowdry and Steinberg, 1975). Estimates indicate a growth rate of 30% since 1975. This figure does not include many county, city, and state health units that are not certified to participate in the Medicare program. Through April 1976, some 200 applications for accreditation had been reviewed by the National League for Nursing, the agency responsible for administration, and the American Public Health Association, (Cowdry and Steinberg, 1976e). Approximately 100 had been accredited by April 1976 under their jointly sponsored program.

Many, if not all, of the certified agencies provide speech pathology services to their patients, either through full-time employees or contract practitioners on a fee-for-service basis.

Types of Home Care Agencies

The Social Security Administration, Bureau of Health Insurance, categorizes home health agencies into the following groups: Visiting Nurse Association - VNA; Combination (official and voluntary agency) - COMB; Official (health department) - OFF; Rehabilitation - REHB; Hospital-based - HOSP; Extended Care Facility - ECF; Proprietary -PROP; and other - OTH. Of the 2,247 certified agencies in 1975, approximately 60% are administered by official health departments,

25% by visiting nurse associations, and 8% by hospitals. The remaining 7% of the programs are operated by combined government and voluntary agencies, prepaid health plans, extended care facilities, rehabilitation agencies, or private independent agencies established for this purpose. Whatever the organizational base, the central administration aids the physician by efficient delivery of appropriate services to his patients, and it assumes the responsibility for smooth coordination of services and for quality control.

The organizational base and structure determines the character and scope of an agency. Hospital-based programs differ greatly in character and scope from community, official, and proprietary agencies. Steinberg (Cowdry and Steinberg, 1971) maintains a more favorable posture for home health services that are hospital sponsored, for such reasons as that the various professional services of the hospital can be made available to the homebound patient. If necessary, the patient can be hospitalized more readily if the home care service is a hospital department. Also, physicians may utilize the home care program more frequently if it is a part of the institution in which they spend the greater part of their professional time. Hospital home care can furnish drugs through the hospital pharmacy and assures a patient a bed at any time, should rehospitalization be required. Sickroom equipment that is either owned by the hospital or rented from an outside agency can be provided for the patient. Specialists in all fields of medicine, dentists, and rehabilitation specialists may see patients at home unless diagnostic or treatment procedures require the use of nontransportable equipment.

Community-based programs administered by county health departments, visiting nurse associations, and some independent agencies often emphasize home nursing, home health aid, and homemaker service. Medical care is provided by the patient's personal physician, although a number of agencies, especially the proprietary ones, engage a physician full time or part time as the Medical Director of the program. If full time, the director may provide medical care to patients; however, the medical care of the patient usually is delivered by the patient's personal physician. In a part-time capacity, the physician director serves as an advisor to the professional personnel of the agency, i.e., nurses, social workers, and speech pathologists. He supervises the quality of care and the medical records. He communicates with the patient's attending physician when difficulties arise. He regularly reviews the patient care policies, evaluates the standards for patient care, and establishes ethical, professional, and medical practices of the agency (Cowdry and Steinberg, 1976c).

Community-based programs include a greater proportion of short-term patients who are using the service while recovering from an acute illness or injury (Cowdry and Steinberg, 1971). Such programs also tend to have more referrals made directly from home than from a hospital. Many may stress the home nursing and fail to provide needed rehabilitation services. However, this situation has improved significantly in recent years after amendments were enacted to Title XVIII of Medicare, requiring facilities to provide the full array of needed services or otherwise not accept the patient for care.

Few home health agencies employ full-time speech pathologists. Those that do are generally the independent proprietary agencies or health department units. Most home health agencies provide all rehabilitative services, including speech pathology, under contract arrangements. Due to a noncompetitive salary scale, 95% of the case load is geriatric, too much of the professional's time is spent in travel, organizational structure precludes professional independence, paper work is prohibitive, and opportunity for advancement is lacking.

Speech pathology programs can be established in home health agencies to circumvent all of these problems, pay their own way, provide good salaries and fringe benefits, create a challenging area of direct service to patients, and stimulate research and professional growth. The first home health agency to be certified to participate in Medicare has had a full-time speech pathology program for almost ten years. In October 1976, it became the first private agency to be accredited by the National League for Nursing and the American Public Health Association. The speech pathology department was accredited under full standards of the American Speech and Hearing Association (Cowdry and Steinberg, 1976b).

Organization and Administration

Home health agencies must have legal authority to operate in the state in which they are located. This is usually accomplished through a charter issued after presentation of Articles of Incorporation to the Secretary of State. Again, this applies more specifically to proprietary agencies then to county or state health department units. The agency should have a stated purpose for its existence, usually found in its corporation Constitution and by-laws.

The legally constituted governing body of an agency is the Board of Directors, who assume full authority and responsibility for the operation of the agency. The Board of Directors may be stockholders and serve as officers of the agency.

The Board of Directors appoints an Advisory Board, which is a group of professional people in the community who advise the agency on professional matters. For example, one such board is composed of 16 members, including medical doctors in private practice, a speech pathologist from the local hospital, a certified public accountant, a medical social worker, the agency administrator, and others. Advisory Board members serve a three-year term. The Board of Directors also appoints an administrator (Executive Director) who has the authority by delegation to oversee the management and fiscal affairs of an agency.

A medical director and sometimes a director of professional services are appointed and given authority by delegation to direct and supervise the skilled nursing and rehabilitative services of the agency. Herein lies a most difficult ethical barrier to speech pathologists. Speech pathologists have traditionally been independent professionals who direct and supervise their own services and are responsible administratively to the agency administrator. The American Speech and Hearing Association and the American Academy of Private Practice in Speech Pathology and Audiology continue to maintain and support the independent role of the speech pathologist. It would therefore be inappropriate for a speech pathologist to work in an organizational setting under individuals who direct and supervise his professional services but who are untrained in speech pathology and audiology. Speech pathologists must insist upon professional independence within the organization but may come under the fiscal and administrative direction of the agency.

Another reason some agencies use contract personnel is that greater professional control can be exercised by other specialists, usually nursing personnel, when full-time speech pathologists are not employed. These nurses may be holding positions that would be more appropriately held by speech pathologists. Education and change are slow processes, but they can occur with a determined, positive, ethical attitude toward the profession, the services speech pathologists provide, and the organizations for whom speech pathology services are provided.

Some agencies realize the need for directors of the various disciplines in their health care delivery system and employ a director of nursing, a director of physical therapy, and a director of speech pathology, engaging a physician to advise the group. This is the preferred organizational structure for the professional areas, the same as would be found in a hospital organizational structure. Each director is responsible administratively to the Agency administrator (Executive Director).

Rehabilitation at Home

While home care, for many patients, offers an alternative to institutionalization, concerns exist regarding its cost-effectiveness and quality. Proponents of home care maintain that home health care can be provided at less cost than care in a hospital or nursing facility, and that its availability and use will reduce the demand for expensive institutional services. Cost-effectiveness may be defined to mean that the cost of a certain way of accomplishing a task is appropriately related to the total social benefits and costs.   In other words, judgements are made not simply on the basis of direct costs, but also on the overall value of the results achieved.

Studies indicate no consensus on the elements necessary for comparison between home care and other forms of care, or to account for differences in the level and intensity of services provided, or for the cost impact on the health, demographic, social, and economic characteristics of the populations served. Equally important, there has been little attempt to consider the effect of an individual's functional status on the cost of care (Cowdry and Steinberg, 1976a).   Most studies are retrospective analyses of the cost of home visits and services, and estimates of the numbers and costs of inpatient days saved as a result of home care.   There has been little in-depth analysis of elements, other than unit (visit or service) costs, aimed at answering the question: "What does it cost to take care of this person at home, in terms of total service, support, and living costs?" (Cowdry and Steinberg, 1971).

Our own data suggest that for many patients, needed services cost less when delivered at home, because often a patient is routinely charged for equipment in hospitals, whether he uses it or not. Also, families assume the care of the patient that aides and nurses render in an institutional setting. However, the cost of speech pathology services delivered in the home is considerably more than those delivered in a private office or clinic for two major reasons. First, patients are always seen on a one-to-one basis in the home, whereas in a clinic or

office a patient can be worked into small
groups. Second, a portion of the professional's time is spent in driving from one
patient to another. The fact remains, however, that regardless of increased costs,
some patients need the services and can
benefit from treatment at home before they
are able to go routinely to a clinic or
practitioner's office.

The treatment goal for patients under-
going rehabilitation is an increase of independence in self-care, ambulation, and communication. This category includes primarily
stroke patients who have been discharged from
inpatient rehabilitation programs in which
they have not reached maximum potential.
Many elderly patients remain poorly motivated
as long as they are in a hospital environment. They are confused by the institutional
setting and by the many nurses and specialists who demand physical effort and mental
concentration. Once they return home, rehabilitative activities generally become more
meaningful, and, subsequently, motivation and
cooperation improve. (Further discussion is
given to specific communication goals and
types of patients in another section of this
chapter.) Definite goals should be established for each patient and understood by all
who attend him. Objectives and achievements
should be reviewed periodically, and home
treatment should be discontinued when the
goals have been achieved or when a reasonable
trial period has proved them to be unachiev-
able.

The assurance of high quality care in
the home is equally important. This can be
achieved through activities and programs
intended to assure quality of care, such as
educational in-service programs, and through
components designed to remedy identified
deficiencies in quality, such as peer or

utilization review and the development of standards of care in terms of patient outcome. Supervision is basic to the provision of higher quality care in the home. The professional who establishes the care plan should provide the supervision; thus, a speech pathologist should supervise other speech pathologists. Supervision should include direct observation with patients, on occasion, as well as staff reporting and record review.

Frequent physician monitoring by a patients's personal physician is suggested, especially for elderly patients with multiple diseases. For example, stress of treatment may precipitate complications. The physician approves plans of treatment by other professionals, such as speech pathologists, in relation to the patient's overall rehabilitation potential and the total care of the patient. Monitoring in no way suggests immediate supervision of professionals such as audiologists, speech pathologists, and psychologists. However telephone and written communication by other professionals to the physician can provide him with valuable information as he sees the patient for treatment.

Highly qualified personnel can assure quality of services perhaps more than any other single factor. Home health agencies should employ or contract only speech pathologists who have at least the minimum qualifications of a masters degree, a state license (where applicable), and the Certificate of Clinical Competence granted by the American Speech and Hearing Association. No one can guarantee high quality except the person actually performing the care, and while a license in and of itself does not necessarily promote quality it can be revoked therefore preventing an incompetent individual from practicing.

Personnel

Earlier, both full-time and contract speech pathologists were mentioned in connection with the various types of agencies and according to the size and types of services offered by the home health agency. Here, greater detail is given to the agency-employed speech pathologist and contract private practitioners.

The speech pathologists employed by a home health agency can expect a fair salary, a transportation allowance, and whatever fringe benefits are provided other full-time employees. The contract speech patholgist is given a fee for service; that is, an agreed upon amount per visit. Usually the agency reimburses at one half of the rate charged. For example, if the agency charges $35.00 per visit, the contract speech pathologist receives between $15 and $20 per visit. Most agencies charge a given rate for any service provided, regardless of the time or discipline involved. Thus, a ten-minute nursing visit costs the same as a 30-minute speech pathology visit. Some agencies, but very few, agree to bill for the speech pathologist for 5% or 10%; thus, the speech pathologist may retain the greater portion of the rate charged per visit.

The agency-employed speech pathologist establishes a program that evaluates, habilitates, and coordinates care of patients with speech and language impairments whether these arise from physiological or neurological disturbances and/or both. Psychologically based speech and language problems are referred to other agencies.

Contract speech pathologists evaluate and habilitate patients with communication problems; however, the program is often planned, directed, and supervised by someone who may or may not be a speech pathologist. Agencies are seldom willing to pay the contract individual for professional time to plan and consult with other professionals on a routine basis. Therefore, a nurse generally plans and directs all of the areas of professional service. This arrangement is completely unacceptable professionally to the speech pathologist and should be discouraged.

Contract individuals can make a choice in the amount of travel they are willing to do and the geographical areas in which they wish to deliver services, while a salaried speech pathologist may have to travel an entire metropolitan area if the case load is small. Travel can be reduced by dividing a metropolitan area between a full-time staff speech pathologist and contract staff who are willing to see patients in limited areas. Diagnostic and treatment materials are provided by the agency for the salaried speech pathologist, while the contract practitioner must provide his own diagnostic and treatment materials to be used with patients.

The contract speech pathologist must carry and furnish evidence of adequate malpractice insurance while the salaried speech pathologist is covered under an agency's umbrella policy covering all professionals providing direct care to patients. This writer strongly suggests that all speech pathologists providing direct services to patients carry malpractice insurance in addition to that provided by an agency.

Both salaried and contract speech pathologists should be provided an adequate orientation to a home care agency. The orienta-

tion is more detailed in areas such as employee benefits and personnel policies for
the salaried speech pathologist than for
contract staff members. However, contract
staff members should be thoroughly acquainted
with the types of patients, Medicare coverage
and regulations, other professional services
provided by the agency, and all forms and
procedures for proper documentation of patient records. Generally, the duties and
responsibilities for patient care, coordination of services, and documentation of records for contract staff are identical with
those of salaried staff (Cowdry and
Steinberg, 1976b).

Contract staff and salaried speech
pathologists need excellent credentials and
professional experience in specific areas.
Under Medicare the minimum credential is a
"masters degree and in the process of obtaining the Certificate of Clinical Competence"
(Cowdry and Steinberg). Many states have a
state licensure law, and the license is a
requirement to treat patients in those
states. Work experience is needed especially
in the area of speech and language for stroke
patients, laryngectomees, and patients with
Parkinson's disease and multiple and lateral
sclerosis. Administrative and supervisory.
training is also essential.

With many speech pathologists needing
work settings to complete their clinical
fellowship year, home care agencies are often
requested to provide an affiliation and the
supervised training. The dilemma of providing supervision of a clinical fellow is
reimbursement, for the home visit only covers
one clinician. The fellow obtains training
with only a limited age group and type of
communicatively impaired individual, primarily patients age 65 and older who are
stroke victims. On the positive side, speech

pathologists who prefer working with this population usually apply. The director of the program can stress certain areas of their training for the home care setting, especially in the areas of record keeping and membership on the multidisciplinary team. The speech pathology program's in-service education program can be directed to increase skills in administrative tasks and supervision. Staff in-service meetings may be scheduled once a month and deal with supervision for several sessions. Here again, differences arise; the contract staff is encouraged to attend such meetings but is not reimbursed for the time spent at them, while the salaried staff is being paid for their time. Some well-planned public relations and motivation techniques are often required to get private practitioners to see the overall value to them and the agency in attending such meetings. One sure way is to have such items listed in the contract. In our ten-year program, the contract staff has been outstanding in participating in in-service activities, patient progress review meetings, and utilization review. As long as both salaried and contract staff members thoroughly understand from the outset what is expected and are treated with a sense of fairness when changes are necessary, a program will be successful and the lack of cooperation minimal. One of our present contract staff members was our affiliate clinical fellow in 1974-75 and has remained with us. She is dependable and can function above average in any area of the department when called upon.

A major advantage of contract staff to the speech pathology program is that during periods when the case load is low, payment is not made to nonutilized personnel. If speech pathologists are salaried employees, they are paid their salary regardless of the case load.

Another aspect to be considered in the use of contract speech pathologists is the length of time a patient is to be treated. Some agencies maintain that contract staff members see their patients for excessive lengths of time. This need not be a problem if personnel have been properly indoctrinated. Education is the key. The speech pathologist must review and note the length of treatment of each patient in terms of his stated potential and whether or not progress has been made.

Reacquisition of communication skills can be very slow for some patients; therefore, it is the speech pathologist's duty to provide information to other health team personnel, fiscal intermediaries, private health insurance carriers, and the consumers of speech pathology services about the types of disorders, the potential for rehabilitation, and the estimated times for reacquisition to occur. Since 99% of the speech cases in home care settings are stroke patients with concomitant speech and language reductions, speech and language programs rarely should exceed a 6 to 8 month period of treatment. This does not mean that many patients would not continue to benefit from treatment, but rather that in this amount of time, the patient will have achieved his greatest amount of gain and family members will have been taught a program of speech and language stimulation that they can continue. Also, the patient is able now to go to a clinic, hospital, or practitioner's office for continued treatment. Certainly not all stroke patients should be treated for a 6 to 8 month period of time. Many patients are seen only one time for an evaluation. Then, because of the patient's age, severe impairment, poor prognosis for improvement, and, sometimes, poor home environment for treatment, speech pathology is not recommended or is delayed until a patient is more stable. Other patients can achieve a limited communication system in the 6 to 8 month treatment period. They would not be considered conversationally adequate but they can communicate needs, wants, and intent through a verbal-gesture-written system. Still others achieve con-versational adequacy in the above-mentioned time period.

Again, patients vary in potential, rate of progress, and, of course, elegibility for benefits, and all of these factors must be considered in determining the treatment time. The speech pathologist should document and pursue his professional opinion and judgement in these matters. Speech pathologists and audiologists are the experts in communication skills and behavior. It is also their task to let others know that they know what they are doing. It often means added work, writ-ing letters of explanation, questioning, and requiring of others their rationale for opposition. However, this process of educa-tion benefits everyone: the patient who needs treatment, the physician who needs help with his patient, and those who determine payment for speech pathology services.

Whether speech pathologists are salaried or contracted by a home agency, they must be prepared to provide many people with informa-tion about what they do and why. If educa-tion is they key, documentation is the lock. The patient's record must reflect what treat-ment is being given by the speech patholo-gist, why the treatment is being given, what the patient's reaction is to the treatment measures, and the justification for continua-tion or termination of treatment. When this is done in a fair, open minded, cautious,

professional manner, there will be little if
any justification for agencies to say contract speech pathologists tend to prolong
treatment excessively.

Duties and Responsibilities

The speech pathologist who is salaried
by a home care agency and who is the director
of the speech pathology department within an
agency has more numerous and comprehensive
duties and responsibilities. The director
must identify and evaluate present and potential needs and resources both in relation to
the community's communicatively handicapped
and to agency policies and procedures. For
example, do geographic boundaries of the
agency preclude speech pathology services to
some groups? Do policies of the agency
regarding high-risk danger areas preclude
services to some? Does the practice of using
only contract staff insure timely and needed
care for patients? The director of the
speech pathology program must work within the
policies and procedures of the agency and
make an effort to change those policies and
procedures when change is in the best interest of communicatively impaired patients.

The director assists in the development
of policies, programs, and functions of the
agency relating to patient care, medical, and
other health care personnel. Patient care
policies for the communicatively impaired may
be reviewed by the agency medical director,
but the policies, practices, and standards
should be planned, directed, and implemented
by the person in charge of the speech pathology program. Supervision and evaluation of
staff speech pathologists are provided by the
director through direct observation, record
review, and individual conference.

The speech pathology director plans, organizes, and assists in providing student educational experiences and affiliations for training programs in the community. These may include speech pathology clinical practice and observational experiences for physical therapists, nurses, and social workers (Cowdry and Steinberg, 1976d).

Staff development activities are planned by the program director. In addition to the agency in-service meetings, workshops, graduate classes, conferences, and conventions are scheduled as a part of continuing education. All staff speech pathologists are encouraged to attend at least the state and national meetings of their professional organizations. A detailed record is kept in the employee's or contract practitioner's file and a copy is submitted to the agency administrator who maintains a continuing education record on all personnel.

The speech pathology director should be a permanent member of the Committee for Periodic Review of Patient Progress and the Utilization Review Committee. The director should also attend the interdisciplinary staff conference conducted by the Agency Administrator, and the bimonthly Advisory Board meetings.

The department budget is planned by the director and submitted to the agency administrator for approval. In addition, the director usually carries a case load of patients equal to that of other staff speech pathologists. However, the case load may be reduced at particular times of unusual activity in the agency. For example, during the months of preparation for accreditation and the agency's annual evaluation, more time is spent in those activities and, of a necessity, fewer patients are seen by the program

director. Few home care speech pathology
programs develop to the point of using a
full-time director. In this writer's opinion, there is also a professional need for
the person who administers and supervises
care of patients provided by others to personally continue, to some degree, to provide
patient care. Strong exception is taken to
persons of any discipline in home care agencies who determine whether or not the care
given is of quality, and who evaluate those
delivering the care, when they themselves
often have not seen a patient in years,
sometimes not since training days. In such
instances the words supervision, evaluation,
peer review, and quality are misused. If the
director provides direct patient care, observation of staff (other than clinical fellows)
can be reduced by having staff members, on
occasion, see those patients that are usually
seen by the director. The feedback in terms
of reporting by the staff speech pathologist,
the patient, and the patient's family gives
great insight into the skills, rapport, and
dependability of the clinician.

Perhaps of all the duties of the director of the speech pathology program, consultation and coordination of patient care can
be most crucial. This means informing the
patient's personal physician of any changes
in care plans and advising other health care
personnel (nurses, physical therapists, and
social workers) of those changes. Changes in
the care plan are always documented in the
medical record, often by the director since
he has immediate access to the record.

As stated earlier, duties and responsibilities of staff speech pathologists, whether contract or salaried, are identical.
Upon referral and physician request (order),
which is usually stated "evaluate and treat
as needed," they evaluate the patient's

speech, hearing, and language skills. The individual speech pathologist selects and administers whatever diagnostic tests are deemed necessary. Recently some intermediaries moved to require that every stroke patient seen for speech pathology services be administered the Porch Index of Communicative Ability and that repeat tests be administered every 60 days prior to additional coverage being granted. Such universality of a specific test instrument is discouraged. The Porch test is an excellent tool for many patients but not for all. Each clinician should have several tests available in his or her clinical materials. (A discussion of the evaluation and care plan and the elements required follows in another section.)

Once the evaluation is made, the speech pathologist who evaluated the patient establishes a written care plan, a copy of which is sent to the patient's physician for his review and signature. It is returned to the agency and becomes a part of the patient's medical record.

Individual speech pathologists must maintain adequate clincial records on patients; generally, a daily progress note, 30- to 60-day progress reports, and discharge summaries. Again, these will be discussed further under the section "clinical or medical record."

Each speech pathologist plans and provides the rehabilitative services to implement the care plan established. These services are coordinated with the services of other health team members, most often the home health aide and the physical therapist. The time of day, the days on which each is to provide care, and the ways each can assist one another are most important. The speech pathologist can suggest ways for the physical therapist to encourage and stimulate speech during his exercise program. The home health aide can often be used just as a member of the family would in practice drills, especially tactile and flexibility exercises of the oral musculature. If a home health aide is utilized in practice drills, he or she should be supervised routinely in these activities by the qualified speech pathologist. Also, the aide's visit can never be substituted for a visit by the speech pathologist. The aide simply uses a portion of his or her scheduled time with the patient to review and practice drills the speech pathologist has suggested. Aides often see patients daily, whereas the speech pathologist sees the patient two to three times a week. Therefore, proper use of the aide can enhance a patient's speech and language program. This is the only way supportive personnel should be utilized in the home.

Staff speech pathologists are expected to use community resources and other agency personnel by proper referral. For example, should a patient's status change so that he is no longer homebound and unable to use the outpatient speech pathology services of the agency, referral should be made to another practitioner or to a community clinic. Patients are often in need of medical equipment, and the speech pathologist should refer such patients to the physical therapist, who obtains the equipment from a local supplier.

Continuing education has become standard in most professional areas in the last ten years. Staff speech pathologists are required to keep up to date on speech, hearing, language, research, and legislation and regulations that affect their services. They must submit evidence annually of attendance at professional conferences, workshops, and

conventions, and should attend those scheduled in-service meetings deemed appropriate.

Each speech pathologist participates in
a systematic plan for review of patient
treatment and progress, which may include
attendance at meetings of the Periodic Review
of Patient Progress Committee held once a
week and the Utilization Review Committee
held once a month. Every 30 days each patient is reviewed by conference or telephone
with the speech pathology director.

Types of Patients

Earlier, the types of patients seen in
home care settings were mentioned as aphasic,
those with Parkinsons disease or multiple and
lateral sclerosis, and laryngectomees. These
disorders occur more frequently in the elderly and are covered by Medicare and private
insurance plans which contain a home care
clause. This coverage is for elderly patients who are unable to routinely make trips
to clinics, physicians' offices, and community clinics.

Aphasia and its correlates account for
the majority of speech pathology patients
seen in the home. Despite divergent points
of view about the nature of aphasia, aphasio-
logists are in agreement that the underlying
cause of aphasia is a physiological distur-
bance secondary to anatomical change result-
ing from brain damage of the dominant (usually left) hemisphere (Travis, 1971). Although aphasic individuals all have incurred
brain damage, this does not imply that all
persons who have incurred brain damage, even
to the dominant hemisphere, become aphasic.

The possible causes of cerebral damage
with which aphasic disturbances are associ-

ated are many and varied. They include direct trauma by externally applied force, tumors, cerebral vascular lesions (embolisms, thromboses, aneurysms, hemorrhages), infectious diseases affecting brain tissue, and degenerative diseases invading the brain. Of these factors the vascular distrubances, embolisms, hemorrhages, and thromboses are the most frequent etiological associates and account for the patients most frequently seen in home settings by speech pathologists.

Cerebral dominance, laterality, and language functions are important in any discussion of aphasia. The intent here is to indicate only that there is agreement among those who have spent considerable time in research (Penfield and Roberts, 1959, p. 102; Russell and Espir, 1961, p. 1970; Osgood and Miron, 1964, p. 49; and Goodglass and Quadfasel, 1954), as to the hemisphere of involvement, the relation of involvement to handedness, and the localization of function within the dominant hemisphere. Most wounds or lesions causing aphasia are almost always on the left cerebral hemisphere. Left cerebral dominance therefore is almost invariable. Aphasia is rarely associated with right cerebral hemisphere damage. There is about a 10% incidence of aphasia in right-handed persons following right cerebral insult and about a 20%-30% incidence in left-handed patients.

Eisenson (Travis, 1971) suggests that right cerebral damage may have implications for language functioning when such functioning is related to high-level intellectual processes. Skills needed in the use of abstract words were found to show the greatest deviations. There also appears to be an intensity of aphasic symptoms in lesions involving the fronto-parietal-temporal and parieto-temporal-occipital regions; thus, a variety of disturbances in fluency, naming, repetition, reading, and writing occur in three major areas of the cerebral cortex (Travis, 1971). It is worth noting that there also seems to be a high degree of disturbances for verbal comprehension associated with lesions of the temporal and parietal regions. The referring phsyician will often indicate to the speech pathologist the site of lesion.

Our own observation and treatment of home-bound aphasic patients suggests that most show some degree of comprehension and intellectual impairment as well as personality modifications. These modifications are brought about by the brain lesions, which have the effect of reducing the patient's capacity to make the necessary adjustments to control undesirable behavior traits such as rigidity, concretism, withdrawal, agressiveness, and hostility. One must remember that an aphasic patient has a personality that is modified by lesions of the cortex and that the impairments become directly and indirectly associated with it. Aphasia produces disruption and the need for reorganization. The preaphasic personality greatly determines what the patient will become.

There is still opposition in many quarters to treatment of aphasics, especially if they are older persons. Our position is that age is immaterial and treatment depends on residual abilities and the objective potential to restore the person to as close to his premorbid status as possible. Emphasis of rehabilitation is on the total person, where speech and language are important aspects but not the sole purpose for treatment. The ultimate goal, of course, is to help the patient find some purpose in life and to achieve acceptance by society, his family, and, in some cases, his fellow workers;

whether he talks or not, the goal is to assist him in gaining a communication system.

Treatment should be initiated at the earliest possible date after onset of cerebral insult. Our experience with aphasics suggests a poor prognosis if the patient is unable to use some auditory input, demonstrated through responses of motor acts, to carry out some simple commands. If he can demonstrate some comprehension, integration, and follow-through, treatment is warranted. Self correction is another indicator of potential for treatment. If a patient is unaware of errors and persists in this unawareness when his attention is directed to it, prognosis for improvement is poor.

Treatment procedures per se will not be detailed. Techniques should allow for the patient's perseverance, concretism, emotional and psychological state, learning characteristics, and reinforcement through reward. Aphasic patients have greater difficulty in learning tasks and are variable in performance; that is, they are inconsistent.

The basic principles which govern the language learning of normal persons, adults as well as children, also hold true for aphasics. Associations are strengthened if they are rewarded. For the adult, usually an indication of "a right response" is sufficient reward. If information and insight can be added to or become integral characteristics of the reward, learning progresses more smoothly and reliably. Learning situations which have an objective, meaningful, and significant goal for the patient, help to motivate and direct the relearning. Remember, for the aphasic, the association areas are impaired or injured and the sensory and neuromotor mechanisms may also be impaired. Residuals of established habits and old plans may interfere with the establishment of new strategies and techniques for learning. Some associations do come back spontaneously for the aphasic, and hence he may hope that spontaneous recovery will continue. This hope may, and frequently does, interfere with voluntary efforts at relearning. Original approaches to learning should be used if the speech pathologist can determine the original way the patient learned content; for example in writing, whether the patient learned manuscript before cursive writing. The patient may be aided initially by having him use manuscript. Handedness is usually changed and is generally accomplished in three or four weeks. Most patients will want to achieve a legible signature.

Our approach to stimulation for most patients is multimodal, using visual, auditory, and tactual pathways. If a patient is unable to use one or the other, of course it is not used; however, all sensory pathways provide cues, and the more each can be utilized, the more linguistic information the patient will have.

Treatment techniques must include, for those who need them, activities for agnosias, reading disturbances (alexia), auditory imperceptions, apraxias, writing (agraphia), paraphasia, word finding difficulty (anomia), and arithmetic problems (acalculia). For specific activities in each category the reader is referred to Speech Disorders: Aphasia, Apraxia and Agnosia by Brain, R. (1961), and The Handbook of Speech Pathology and Audiology edited by Travis, Lee E. (1971).

Some laryngectomees are seen by the speech pathologist in the home setting. The surgeon decides if there is sufficient residual tissue for the patient to learn esopha-

geal speech. There also may be a physical
condition in which a patient is not physically strong enough to attempt the practice
of achieving sound. In some cases, an artificial larynx is obtained immediately. The
artificial larynx is the one reimbursable
prosthesis that the speech pathologist can
obtain for patients under Medicare. Generally, the patient is given approximately ten
sessions to achieve fairly good sound and
control of inhalation and exhalation. Loudness and preciseness of articulation are
variable with the individual patient. Most
patients can achieve some use of the electro-
larynx during the first session. The laryn-
gectomee is seldom seen for more than 10 to
18 speech sessions. Snidecor gives an excellent presentation in the Travis book (1971),
including esophageal speech techniques.

Degenerative diseases of the brain include Parkinsonism, pseudo-bulbar palsy, and
multiple and lateral sclerosis. For patients
with these diseases, reversal of the disorder
and improvement in speech skills is impossible; however, with some modern medication,
the degenerative processes are slowed and
sometimes contained. The home care speech
pathologist is sometimes requested to see
these patients. Providing information to the
patient and his family is most beneficial.
Establishing a maintenance program of exercises to maintain vocal inflections, tone,
and rate of speech is important. An exercise
program for the oral musculature in terms of
mastication as well as speech can encourage
and benefit many of these patients. Above
all, the emotional support and counseling of
the patient and family alleviates much of the
fear and hostile feelings. Patients generally are seen twice a week for a 30-day
period, or for about ten sessions.

Program and Service Evaluation

A home health agency must initate ways of evaluating the agency's total program and service areas. This is usually accomplished through the committees of which the speech pathologist is a member.

First is the Annual Evaluation Committee. The annual evaluation is a major function of the Agency Advisory Board. For the purpose of evaluation, the Advisory Board is divided into three subcommittees: the medical subcommittee, the personnel subcommittee, and the financial subcommittee.

The agency program evaluation is primarily the responsibility of the medical subcommittee. The purpose of the medical subcommittee is to ascertain whether the overall philosophy, approach, quality, and quantity of health care services provided by the agency is in keeping with the stated philosophy, goals, and program objectives. It is also the purpose of the medical subcommittee to determine whether the philosophy and objectives as stated by all disciplines are implemented at the patient level.

In order to meet these two overall aims, a selective review of patients' clinical records, as well as a survey of the referring physician and patient population through questionnaires, is conducted by the members of the medical subcommittee.

This subcommittee institutes a mailing of an evaluation form to all active patients and the attending physicians of patients discharged during the three-month period prior to the study, in order to secure an evaluation of patient care provided by the agency.

The medical subcommittee, in beginning the self-evaluation study of the agency program, first establishes objectives to be used as the criteria for review of services which deal directly with patient care. The following are the objectives established by this committee for the last evaluation.

To determine:

1.   If the agency is fulfilling its obligation to the community by providing home care for maximum rehabilitation within the individual limitations in a reasonable length of time.

2.   If the services offered by the agency to referred patients are provided as quickly as possible in order to meet the needs of the physician, patient, and family.

3.   If the agency is meeting specific health needs of selected patients for home care.

4.   The quality of care the agency is providing to the patient population.

5.   Whether the established policies regarding professional health care, as stated in the philosophy and objectives of the agency, are implemented at the patient level.

6.   If the care provided by each service is utilized appropriately and sufficiently.

7.   The sentiments of the physicians and consumers regarding care provided by the agency.

8.   If care rendered by the agency is instrumental in the rehabilitation of the patient.

9.   The physical, social, emotional, and rehabilitation profile of the typical patient.

10.   If the accepted agency policies regarding admission and discharge of patients are reflected in the agency's records.

11.   The number of patients requiring additional services beyond the extent of Medicare.

12.   That, upon discharge from the agency, continued care is established for the patient as needed.

13.   That the confidentiality between the patient and his physician is maintained.

14.   That the attending physician alone is the person in charge of patient care and is totally respected by agency personnel in providing medical services.

Another method of evaluating services is the utilization review. The Utilization Review Committee is a method of systematic evaluation used to improve patient care and to ensure the appropriate use of services rendered to individuals, families, and the community. The process produces information for program evaluation on an ongoing basis. It also produces information for planning for staff development; both strengths and weaknesses are identified so that further action can be taken based on these. The Utilization Review Committee meets regularly and reviews

a ten percent sampling of active, closed, and
rejected charts.

A review form is developed by the agency
for use by the Utilization Review Committee.
In Utilization Review Committee meetings,
each committee member reviews individual
charts, using the designated review form.
During the review process, the reviewer
determines if:

1. The individual patient's needs (as
    reflected in the documented charts)
    were met by the agency services.

2. The services were adequate in
    range, intensity, and duration.

3. The services are coordinated and
    involve appropriate team members
    both within and outside the agency.

4. Continuity of patient care is
    provided both within and outside
    the agency.

5. Appropriate utilization of commun-
    ity resources is provided.

Following the individual record review,
a summary of the findings is presented to the
committee by each reviewer. The committee as
a whole prepares a report of its findings and
recommendations as to strengths and weaknesses. The statistical data regarding
deficiencies in chart documentation are
tabulated and totaled per month and cumula-
tively.

A third evaluation measure in most
agencies is the Review of Patient Progress
Committee. This committee is a multidisciplinary committee with representatives from
all service areas. The committee meets three

to four times a month and is chaired by the medical director. Each patient's care is reviewed every 30 to 60 days. If there are unusual problems or occurrences, the patient's case may be presented to the committee at any time. A team member is responsible for presenting to the committee information about type of care being given, patient progress, and future plans. All aspects of care received, i.e., nursing, speech pathology, nutrition, social services, and/or a home health aide are discussed and evaluated. The multidisciplinary team will make recommendations as indicated. Any suggestion or modification of the plan of treatment, which requires a physician's order, is communicated to the patient's physician for his approval prior to any action.

The committee also concerns itself with under- or over-utilization of care and services in relation to the individual patient's needs.

A written progress report is initiated by the appropriate staff member and is completed by the medical director of the committee at the time of the team's conference. The report indicates the committee's evaluation of patient progress, changes in patient care, and/or plans for discharge. A copy of this report is forwarded to the patient's physician. This procedure is, in essence, a record review of patient care and an oral discussion of findings and recommendations.

Peer revew is provided through the director of speech pathology's reviewing patient records and making field visits to observe other speech pathologists. Also, consultation is available from the advisory board member who is a qualified speech pathologist and audiologist. Speech pathology audit committees also serve in a peer review capacity.

Contract speech pathologists may serve at times on any of these committees.

Patient's Medical Record

The patient's medical record is defined as a record which contains sufficient information to identify the patient clearly, to justify his diagnosis and treatment, and to document the results accurately. The purposes of the record are to serve as the basis for planning and continuity of patient care; to provide a means of communication among physicians and any other professionals contributing to the patient's care; to furnish documentary evidence of the patient's course of illness and treatment; to serve as a basis for review, study, and evaluation; to serve in protecting the legal interests of the patient, hospital, and responsible practitioner; and to provide data for use in research and education.

Medical records and their contents are not usually available to the patient himself. The content of the record is usually confidential; however, the patient now has the right to review his records. Home care agencies keep their own records of the care they provide patients in their homes. Most agencies use the more traditional form of medical record; however, some home health agencies have adopted the use of the problem oriented medical record (POMR) (Teuber, 1976).

The problem oriented medical record is one in which the information and conclusions contained in the record are organized to describe each of the patient's problems. The description should include subjective, objective, and significant negative information, discussion, and conclusions, as well as diagnostic and treatment plans with respect to each problem. The POMR was developed by Lawrence Weed, M.D., and has gained increasing acceptance. Initially, it is a little more difficult to get used to because of its formality and organization.

Whatever the type of record system used in a home care agency, the speech pathologist's data become a part of that record system. In most home health agencies, the past medical history and identifying information on patients are obtained by the admissions nurse. The speech pathologist receives a referral form with some of the information, usually enough to make an evaluation.

The evaluation report includes minimal identifying data, diagnosis, type and severity of the communication disorder, tests administered (standardized or nonstandardized), results and interpretations of communicative disorders, prognosis, recommendations, and the signature of the speech pathologist. Testing during the evaluation must include appropriate test instruments, an oral peripheral examination, and a hearing screening. Samples of connected speech are also recommended when possible.

The report of the evaluation itself should be as brief as possible, since a copy goes to intermediaries and physicians. Our experience led us to develop the evaluation shown in Figure 1.

The speech pathology care plan is developed from data obtained during the evaluation. The care plan should include identifying information, the goals and objectives of treatment, the frequency and duration of treatment, modalities to be utilized in treatment (visual, auditory, tactual), and specific activities of treatment. Again, these should be as concise as possible. The care plan shown in Figure 2 has served us well for many years. It is brief, but contains enough information to give a clear picture of the speech pathology treatment provided the patient to all those who review the patient's record, to the patient's physician, and to the fiscal intermediaries.

Progress notes are kept on patients for each visit made by the speech patholgist and are submitted within a five-day period. The notes should include the treatment given during the session, the patient's reaction to the treatment, and any counseling, emotional support, and teaching of aides or families during the session.

When the patient is discharged from speech pathology, a discharge summary is written and attached to the medical record. Again, the patient's physician receives a copy of the summary. Generally, agencies provide the necessary form, which is in triplicate. The summary should briefly state the period of time the patient received treatment, the progress made, and the reason for discharge.

Contracts

Contracts between private practitioners and home health care agencies must be arranged very carefully. The contract must clearly specify the parties involved, demonstrate a purpose for its existence, and enumerate service areas, the fee to be paid, the services the speech pathologist will provide, and the obligations of the agency. The contract should provide a means of renewal and termination. Finally, it must be dated and signed by the agency administrator and the speech pathologist.

If an agency participates in Medicare, the conditions of participation require elements of a contract for service arrangement. Based upon our experience with various intermediaries, including the Bureau of Health Insurance, we have developed the contract shown in Figure 3. Again it has proven most useful.

REFERENCES

Brain R: Speech Disorders: Aphasia, Apraxia, and Agnosia. Washington, D.C., Butterworths, 1961, pp XL

Cowdry EV, Steinberg FU: The Care of the Geriatric Patient: Home Care. C. V. Mosby Company, 1971, pp 384-410

Cowdry EV, Steinberg FU: Home Health Agency, Manual, 2-70, Conditions of Participation, HIM-11 (6-66), Washington, D.C, Department of Health, Education and Welfare, Social Security Administration, 72 pp

Cowdry EV, Steinberg FU: Home Health Care Report, 1976 DHEW Publication No. 76-135. Report on the Regional Public Hearings of the Department of Health, Education and Welfare, Washington, D.C., 1976a, 106 pp

Cowdry EV, Steinberg FU: Home Health Care of Louisiana, Inc., 1976. Accrediation Report for National League for Nursing and the American Public Health Association, 1976b, 605 pp

Cowdry EV, Steinberg FU: Home Health Services of Louisiana, Inc., 1976. Policy and Procedure Manual, 1976c, pp 113, 117-119

Cowdry EV, Steinberg, FU: Home Health Services of Louisiana, Inc., rev. 1976. Speech Pathology Manual, 1976d, 228 pp

Cowdry EV, Steinberg FU: National League for Nursing, Council of Home Health Agencies and Community Health Agencies, 1975. Directory of Home Health Agencies Certified as Medicare Providers. Publication No. 21, 1565, New York, 1975, 109 pp

Cowdry EV, Steinberg FU: Nursing Outlook, 1976. Home Health Agencies and Community Nursing Services Accredited by NLN/APHA. Vol. 24, No. 4, New York, National League for Nursing, April 1976e, pp 1-5

Teuber H: Effects of brain wounds implicating right or left hemisphere in man, in Mountcastle, V. (ed.): Interhemispheric Relations and Cerebral Dominance. Baltimore, The Johns Hopkins Press, 1962, pp 26-41

Teuber H: Staff, Subcommittee on Health and the Environment of the Committee on Interstate and Foreign Commerce, U.S. House of Representatives. A Discursive Dictionary of Health Care, Washington, D.C., U. S. Government Printing Office, 1976, 182 pp

Travis LE, ed.: Handbook of Speech Pathology and Audiology. Englewood Cliffs, New Jersey, Prentice-Hall, 1971, pp 1219-1276

APPENDIX

CHAPTER VII

SPEECH PATHOLOGY EVALUATION

DATE: _____

FROM: _____
      _____

TO: _____
    _____

SUBJECT: Diagnostic Report

Patient Name: _____   Patient Agency No.: _____

Age: _____   Date of Onset: _____

DIAGNOSIS: _____

Type and Severity of Communication Disorder: _____
_____

178

Standardized and Nonstandardized Test Administered: _____

Results and Interpretations of Communicative Disorders: _____

Prognosis: _____

Recommendations: _____

_____
Speech Pathologist

FIGURE 1

179

SPEECH PATHOLOGY CARE PLAN

FROM: _____

TO: _____

SUBJECT: Care Plan

Patient Name: _____   Patient Agency No.: _____

Goals and Objective:

1. Short Term:

2. Long Term: _____

_____

_____

_____

Treatment:

1. Frequency: _____

_____

2. Duration: _____

_____

3. Modalities: _____

_____

4. Activities: _____

_____

FIGURE 2

CONTRACT BETWEEN A SELF-EMPLOYED SPEECH PATHOLOGIST AND AN AGENCY

AGREEMENT BETWEEN

_____, Speech Pathologist

AND

HOME HEALTH SERVICES OF _____ INCORPORATED

This agreement is made and entered into this _____ day of _____, 19 ___, by and between _____, a qualified Speech Pathologist, licensed and/or registered in the State of _____, and Home Health Services of _____, hereinafter referred to as the Agency.

WITNESSETH:

WHEREAS, the Agency has identified a need for Speech Pathology services in the area which it is authorized to serve; and,

WHEREAS, at the present time, the Agency does not have sufficient Speech Pathology services or cannot employ a full-time Speech Pathologist to fulfill the demands; and,

WHEREAS, it is to the Agency's interest, the community's benefit, and the enhancement of patient care to provide Speech Pathology services as herein specified; and,

WHEREAS, _____, Speech Pathologist is prepared to assume the responsibility for providing Speech Pathology services; now therefore,

IT IS AGREED BETWEEN THE AGENCY AND THE SPEECH PATHOLOGIST AS FOLLOWS:

1. The patients are accepted for care only by the Agency.

2. The Speech Pathologist will provide service in the following categories: ___ patient care, ___ teaching, ___ supervision, ___ consultation, ___ policy writing, upon request from appropriate Agency personnel.

3. The services will be provided on a part-time basis.

4. The services shall be provided within the geographic area serviced by the Agency, which includes the Parishes/counties of _____ and _____.

5. The Agency shall pay the Speech Pathologist for services rendered pursuant to this agreement, at a rate of $ _____ per visit. The Speech Pathologist shall keep records and show computation of charges.

6. The Speech Pathologist shall bill the Agency monthly for services rendered during the preceding 30 days and the Agency shall pay all such bills within 15 days.

7. The Speech Pathologist will conform to all applicable Agency policies including personnel qualifications. The duties and responsibilities of the Speech Pathologist are those defined in the Agency policy manual. The Speech Pathologist shall perform his work in accordance with the currently approved methods and practice of his profession and according to the Code of Ethics of his professional association.

8. The speech pathology service provided to the patient will be in response to a request form, and in accordance with a plan established by a physician licensed to practice medicine in the State. Services provided are to be within the scope set forth in the plan and may not be altered by the Agency. Any alteration in the plan of treatment will be between the Speech Pathologist and the referring physician with proper communication to other health personnel involved in the care of the patient. The Speech Pathologist will not accept patients under this agreement without the express approval of the Agency.

9. The Agency shall make available all records and information relevant to the patient for purposes of the services being provided. The Speech Pathologist must maintain records and reports in accordance with the policy of the Agency, including progress notes and observations on the progress of the patient. A daily patient progress note is submitted to the Agency within a five (5) day period. All visits are scheduled by the individual Speech Pathologist. Patient evaluations are written by Speech Pathologists on initial visit and 30 day intervals, copies of same are sent to the attending physician. Initial evaluations are to be written and mailed the same day the patient is seen. A daily summary of services form itemizing Speech Pathologist, contract number, date, day, patient and patient's Agency number is accompanied by the daily progress notes. When deemed necessary by the Agency's Medical Director, the Speech Pathologist will participate in the Agency's Utilization Review and Periodic

Review of Patient Progress. Services provided are controlled by individual

Speech Pathologists to other members of the professional team and evaluated by a

30 day progress report, Periodic Review of Patient Progress Committee (PROPP)

and Utilization Review Committee.

10. The Speech Pathologist will participate in Agency meetings on Patient Care and

will participate in such in-service training sessions conducted by the Agency as

may seem advisable.

11. The Speech Pathologist shall provide a valid certificate of insurance evidencing

that he has adequate professional liability insurance coverage for his services.

12. The Speech Pathologist shall provide the needed equipment unless other arrange-

ments have been agreed upon by the Speech Pathologist and the Agency.

13. This Agreement shall continue and be binding upon the parties hereto from year

to year unless terminated as herein provided. This agreement may be amended by

written consent of both parties and all amendments shall be attached to this

Agreement and made a part thereof.

14. This Agreement may be terminated at any time by either party by the giving of thirty (30) days' written notice of intention to the other party.

_____
Agency Administrator

_____
Speech Pathologist

_____
Date

187

PART III

CHAPTER VIII

CLINICAL ASPECTS OF AUDIOLOGY

Roy C. Rowland, Jr., Ph.D.

Introduction

Audiology has changed considerably over the past decade. Its earlier growth as a federal and state government-supported field in identification, clinical service, and research has slowed, while training programs continue to produce graduates out of proportion to the government's demand. This apparent surplus has created a strong interest (especially among job seekers) in private practice. However, most training programs were, and continue to be, geared to training for the same government services which spawned them. This results in the creation of competent clinicians who are ill-prepared to cope with the stresses and financial insecurity of the private sector of delivery of health services. Ultimately, this situation should prove to be a healthy one for the profession by giving it a stronger base and, through feedback, alteration of training programs to meet the changing needs of audiology. In the interim, a large number of audiologists will enter the private sector with varying degrees of success. It is the purpose of this chapter to enhance the odds in favor of the audiologist by providing some practical guidelines for private practice based upon experience. The Appendix attached to this chapter includes examples of forms used in an independent audiological practice.

The question most often asked of the audiologist already in private practice is usually a variation of the following: "I am an audiologist considering private practice. What do I need to know before I go into practice?" The question, while sincere, is impossible to answer because there is a great deal of missing information that the practicing audiologist needs to know before giving an intelligent answer. For example: What does the person mean by the term audiologist? What is the questioner's academic and experiential background? What does he bring with him in the way of educational and technical skills, aside from the fact that he has something that lets him call himself an audiologist? Also, what does the person mean by the term "considering" private practice? Has he done any real investigating or is he just looking for a job? Is he trying to achieve some goal? Does he want a real change in what he is doing with his life? Is he after extra money? Is he interested in full-time or part-time practice? What is his concept of private practice? Does he mean going into practice with an established ear, nose, and throat center, or is he planning on going it alone? If he is going into a situation where others are already working, is there an existing fee schedule or is he going to have to make one up himself? So, what he needs to know depends in great part on what he already knows, not only about audiology but also about equipment, professional relationships, and sound business practices.

Reasons for Private Practice

One of the most important considerations in establishing a practice is to evaluate why the individual is considering this kind of employment. One needs to examine carefully motives as well as goals to be reached or expectations derived from such a job setting. Since there are both "right" and "wrong" reasons for most decisions, the audiologist should take some time for soul searching as to his particular reasons for entering the private sector. Some of his reasons might include the following:

1. There are no other jobs available. This may seem to be a very pragmatic reason, but alone, it is not sufficient. Success as a practitioner requires more than a forced choice. If this is the primary reason for considering private practice, some thought should be given to temporary employment (full- or part-time) in something else while developing a practice or until the job market improves.

2. The audiologist admires someone who is in private practice. This is laudable, but not predictive of success. The practitioner may serve as a model and sounding board, but not as a reason for entering private practice.

3. The audiologist wants to earn some extra money. It is almost impossible to design a program to accomodate a part-time practice. Space, equipment, and other overhead costs are relatively the same for audiology whether one works 5 or 50 hours a week. Testing one day a week for a physician is not private practice. It is, rather, an employee position.

4. The audiologist wants to earn a lot of money. While the average net income of the person in an established practice may be well above that of some of his colleagues, it

was not always so, and the private
practitioner invests much more time
per net income received.

5.   The audiologist wants to be his own
boss.   Although this is a better
motive than the previous ones, true
independence is elusive.   First,
there is an inverse relationship
between security and independence,
and the audiologist may find himself compromising with medicine as
an employee in order to guarantee
some income.   Second, he will find
that he is closely bound to his
practice, in terms of time, by the
demands of patients and referral
sources.

6.   The concept of patient management
appeals to the audiologist. Theo-
retically, this is one of the best
reasons for considering a private
work environment.   The audiologist
becomes more responsible out of a
necessity to maintain the good will
of his referral sources as well as
the patients themselves.   However,
he will have the problem of determining when, or at what point in
the   diagnostic-habilitation   process, the person becomes his patient, apart from the role of
medicine.

Certainly there are many more reasons why an
audiologist considers private practice, and
perhaps all of them are valid.   The point is
that the more reasons one has for such an
endeavor, the better are the chances for
success.   The audiologist with only one or
two motives would do well to reconsider his
employment goals.

Qualifications for Private Practice

The practice of audiology and the individual engaged in it vary widely throughout the country. Typically, one may think of the audiologist as having a master's degree from an accredited program--one who has completed the clinical fellowship year and holds the Certificate of Clinical Competence. These credentials are certainly basic prerequisites, but they do not necessarily qualify one for private practice.

The American Academy of Private Practice in Speech Pathology and Audiology recommends these basic qualifications, plus either a doctorate and three years' experience or five years experience with the master's degree. The doctorate is not suggested for baseless "snob appeal" as some might think. All of us who have paused in our education between the masters level and the doctorate have some negative attitudes about the value of a Ph.D. The fact that doctoral programs are not more clinically oriented is most unfortunate; however, there are other benefits which accrue to the extended educational process that are valuable to the private practitioner. The most obvious benefit is the use of the title of "doctor," which carries considerable weight with members of other professions, in terms of referral, and with patients, in terms of accepting and following professional advice.

Another very important result of additional education is a deeper understanding of the theoretical basis of auditory function and its impact on human behavior. Most of us have had experiences of supervising and working with individuals at the master's level both before and after completion of the clinical fellowship year (CFY), and we are often disturbed by their inability to explain

their reasons for various procedures other
than to respond with "I was told to do it
that way." Certainly it is possible to gain
the respect and confidence of other professionals and patients without the time and
expense of a doctorate, and the dedicated,
curious student can inquire sufficiently into
auditory theory to enable him to provide
quality service. However, the recommendation
for training beyond the master's degree
remains.

Ideally, the student audiologist should
have had a significant percentage of his
clinical practicum in a private setting.
This is unlikely, however, because of ethical
and legal complications for charging fees for
services performed by students. Some training centers have begun employing private
practitioners to assist in supervising students, and this may be the solution to students' gaining appropriate experience. In
the absence of such a training environment,
an arrangement for employment with a private
audiologist during the CFY is an alternative.
If there is a point to this line of reasoning, it is: One needs private practice
experience before one begins private practice.

Perhaps there is no such thing as a
private practice personality, but there are
some traits which are valuable. These include a sense of humor, an even disposition
or ability to control emotion, salesmanship,
and the ability to work alone. By sense of
humor, I do not mean the improper practice of
deriding patients when talking to other
professionals. Few things are more destruc-
tive to the practitioner than to be recognized as one who makes fun of the impairments
of his patients. The humor required is the
ability to laugh at the frustrations of
private practice. For example, consider a

late arrival to the office due to traffic in
a rainstorm. The secretary is ill. There
are four patients waiting (this is a very
good practice). The first patient is an
angry uncooperative child (complete with a
similarly equipped parent), and the practitioner discovers that he has a dead earphone.
Without humor, and ability to control emotion, a good practice may quickly become
nonexistent.

Selling oneself to patients and referral
sources is something one does everyday in
practice, not only face to face with the
patients, but also in phone conversations and
reports. Therefore, selling experiences in a
variety of environments are worth obtaining
before trying to promote the sale of audiological services.

Audiology in its present state is often
remote and lonely. There are usually few
other professionals in the area, and communication with physicians beyond reporting is
difficult. The private practitioner must be
able to function with this professional
solitude.

Roles in Private Practice

Whether the audiologist is able to
establish an independent practice or works in
a supervised medical setting, he cannot avoid
the role of technician. When the audiologist
performs a series of tests, either on order
or by his own design, his function is technical in nature. For example, performing an
air and bone threshold test and/or a speech
reception-discrimination test is a technical
function. The performance of the test differs significantly from a professional judgement as to which tests are necessary. There
is nothing degrading about functioning as a

technician as long as one realizes that it is only one of several possible roles and not the entire pattern of professional service.

A role that stands much higher in this hierarchy is the clinician level. Here the audiologist makes decisions as to how much testing is required, when to initiate or terminate a procedure, and how to interpret the results in terms of information for medicine or rehabilitation. The clinician "reads" the patient, and, on the basis of written history, verbal exchange, and observation of behavior, constantly adjusts his approach to obtain maximum information with minimum time. Professional efficiency is a major goal of the clinical level.

In addition to deciding upon procedures, performing the tests, and interpreting the results, the audiologist must translate this material into meaningful information for his patient. At this level of advising, the audiologist functions in the role of counselor. Here his job is to provide an honest assessment of the results, explaining the impact of hearing impairment to the patient and his family and urging appropriate techniques, such as amplification and therapy, for remediation.

Occasionally, the audiologist is called upon to assess a situation and provide information that is not directly related to patients. For example, he may be employed by an industry to survey noise and to establish a hearing conservation program for employees. Or, the job might be to establish personnel and equipment guidelines and test techniques for a hearing screening program in a public school. When the audiologist functions in a study-recommendation fashion, he is working as a consultant.

Income as a Private Practitioner

Profit has become a much maligned and misunderstood term in the profession of audiology. Government and nonprofit clinics may have large salaries and expense allowances, and employees may also enjoy holidays, vacation, sick leave, medical coverage, retirement, travel allowances, and other benefits. And yet, because such clinics are legally nonprofit, it is assumed that no profit motive exists in developing fee schedules or deciding which programs will be within the clinic's scope. Profit is nothing more than gross income minus overhead which equals net income. In private practice, profit or net becomes the amount one pays oneself. It can only be determined subsequent to some period of time. Conversely, a nonprofit group accounts for all expenses, including salaries, on an a priori basis.

The private practitioner cannot budget in a futuristic manner. Although some fees lend themselves to time-cost analysis and projection, scheduling variables make many cost projections impractical. For example, although there are 2,080 working hours per year (40 hours x 52 weeks), deductions for holidays, vacations, sick leave, and meetings will reduce this figure to about 1,600 hours. Assuming a conservative overhead of $1,500 per month (secretary, rent, equipment lease, office supplies, telephone, etc.), an annual salary of $20,000 before taxes and without other benefits would indicate an hourly fee schedule of about $25.50. However, if the audiologist charged on that basis, he would fall far below his projection at year's end. There are several reasons for this failure. First, it may take years to build a practice that will occupy the full 40 hours with patients. Second, many people will cancel one or more appointments. Third, many more

will not pay. Therefore, in order to reach
his income goal, the audiologist would have
to charge as much as double his projected
hourly rate. The announcement by a beginning
master's level audiologist that he charges
$50.00 per hour is not likely to be met with
great enthusiasm from other professions.

How then, can fees be designed to provide $50.00 per hour? Part of the answer is
efficiency and the subdividing of test procedures. Many clinics charge on the basis of a
total evaluation (hearing or hearing aid
evaluation, special test battery, ENG, therapy, etc.). Each of those services includes
a variety of procedures. The private practitioner must identify the elements of the
evaluation, the relative sophistication of
knowledge and equipment needed for each
element, and the time involved in order to
price the service. For example, a hearing
evaluation consists of a series of monaural
procedures (air conduction thresholds, bone
conduction thresholds, speech reception
thresholds, speech discrimination tests,
tolerance levels, comfort levels, etc.).
Additionally, pure tone tests may include a
few or several frequencies. By breaking the
examination down, the audiologist can provide
only those services needed to obtain the
necessary information, and can offer the
patient or referral source a cost range
rather than a fixed fee which include
procedures unnecessary to determine the
patient's problem. When asked by a patient
or physician, "What do you charge to test a
child?", the answer could then be "We charge
from $15 to $40." The same principal applies
to other evaluations. Some examples of how
services can be divided are:

	COST
Minimum charge per visit	_____
Air conduction screening (5 frequencies)	_____
Air conduction threshold (frequencies per ear)	_____
Additional frequencies--per ear	_____
Bone conduction threshold-- per ear	_____
Speech reception threshold-- per ear	_____
Speech discrimination--per list	_____
MCL, TL--per ear	_____
Tone decay--per frequency	_____
Bekesy--per test	_____
Stenger	_____
MLB	_____
ABLB	_____
Tympanogram--per ear	_____
Acoustic reflex--per frequency	_____
Occular motor (ENG)	_____
Positional nystagmus testing (ENG)	_____
Caloric (ENG)	_____

This list of possible tests and divisions is by no means complete. The point is that an evaluation consists of many parts. One may need all of them or only a post-surgery monaural air conduction recheck. Most private patients and referral sources will be receptive to a selective procedures schedule with a minimum and maximum fee structure.

In addition to specific fees per test, there are general fees which must be based strictly on time. These fees include therapy or orientation, counseling, consultation, expert witness, and compensation evaluations. Therapy, orientation fees, and counseling fees should be presented in not less than half-hour segments. Consultation fees should be presented for hourly and daily segments. In the event of telephone consultations or

counseling with a patient, a quarter-hour
division is recommended. Accurate date and
time records for telephone work should always
be kept. The audiologist may be asked to
justify such information, and it should be
itemized in office records. Expert witness
service should be charged hourly, including
travel time.

Compensation evaluations were listed in
the general fee category for several reasons.
First, one generally knows in advance that
all routine tests plus some additional objective and nonorganic procedures must be included. Second, an extensive interpretive
report is required. Third, the referral
source will want to know in advance how much
the total charge will be.

Billing Tips

Whether one uses handwritten statements
or computer cards for billing here are some
suggestions which might be helpful in getting
paid for services rendered.

1. Personal notes. Do not pass up an
   opportunity to express appreciation
   to the patient or to the referral
   source for patronage. A handwritten note on the bill expressing
   thanks or pleasure is a simple but
   important gesture.

2. Itemizing. Although one should
   keep an itemized list of the procedures for the record, it is seldom
   necessary to repeat all procedures
   performed on the bill (Medicare,
   Medicaid, and insurance excepted).
   A note on the bill that an itemized
   accounting of services and charges
   is available on request is sufficient.

3. Insurance. The audiologist must make it clear to the patient that the agreement for payment for services is with the patient and not with the insurance company. Offer to assist in recovering payment from the carrier, but explain that such recovery is time-consuming and expensive. It is better to first collect for services and to provide the patient with a signed itemized statement indicating that payment has been made in full. If the patient resists this approach, offer to process the forms, but make an additional charge for the service. Caution: Be certain there is a clearly visible notice stating that there will be a charge of $_____ for filing insurance forms. (See Appendix to this chapter)

4. Forms. Forms and procedures for filing insurance, Medicare, and Medicaid claims have become elaborate and complicated. Request an appointment with representatives of such programs and major medical insurance groups to review preferred methods and forms for filing. This provides a contact to call when there is a problem.

5. Monthly vs. immediate billing. The beginning small practice should probably use an immediate billing method. Billing costs can be reduced by requesting payment from the patient at the time of the testing, but there will be many occasions when this is not practical. Monthly billing has some advantages for bookkeeping, but it

slows cash flow, and too much delay
can reduce the willingness of the
patient to pay for the services.
In the case of slow paying accounts,
the use of stick-on reminders is
helpful. Before turning an account
over to a collection agency, a
telephone call may be in order. It
is better to get some of the money
by compromise than to lose half to
a collection agency or perhaps more
through litigation. Intake forms
will provide some clues as to
whether to insist on payment at the
time of service (unemployed, no
telephone, distant address, etc.).

Space

Professional space is usually rented or
leased on the basis of so much per square
foot per period (monthly or yearly). The
cost varies considerably and choice may be
limited by desirability of a particular
location and availability of a unit of proper
size within the building or complex. Given a
choice, it is financially safer to rent than
to lease. The cost is usually more for
rental, but what appeared to be an excellent
location at first may turn out to be disap-
pointing. Shifts in population density occur
rapidly, and a thriving professional area can
become desolate. Then the long-term lease
becomes a heavy financial liability.

Because space is a costly, recurring
budget item, it must be chosen and used
wisely. The professional must think in terms
of income-producing space versus non-income-
producing space. Most of the income for the
audiologist is produced in the test room.
Therefore, that room should receive first
priority. If the test area is designed and

constructed instead of purchased as a unit,
it can double as a counseling area.

Selection of a waiting or reception area
creates a minor dilemma. Because it falls in
the category of non-income-producing space,
its size needs to be restricted. However, it
is also the place of first impression for the
patient. The best compromise is to keep the
area small (room for four or five persons is
sufficient), but make it attractive, sooth-
ing, and quiet.

Personal office space is the least
essential area. While every professional may
desire something elaborate and impressive,
financial judgement should prevail in keeping
the office simple and reasonable. There will
be an increasing need for file storage, and
allowance for additional cabinets should be
kept in mind.

If the area allows, room and facilities
should be available for at least a refrigera-
tor and coffee facilities. By having both
lunch and refreshments available, the audiologist can more easily extend work time
through the day for himself and for other
staff members. The few minutes saved each
day adds up to a considerable amount of time
over a year's operation.

When selecting space, pay attention to:

1. The general location with respect
    to potential referral sources.

2. Traffic patterns for general acces-
    sibility.

3. Parking facilities.

4. General sound level.

5.   Access to restrooms.

6.   Lavatory facilities.

7.   Electrical load capacity and number
     of outlets.

8.   Heating and air conditioning ser-
     vice and noise level.

Equipment

Sound-Treated Room.   The audiologist spends
most of his time in the control and test room
of the sound-treated area and therefore needs
to plan accordingly.   It is possible to
construct a room that will be adequate for
test purposes (not for research) for about
one-third the cost of a premanufactured metal
room.

     If the area is relatively quiet to begin
with (away from hallways, elevators, heating
and air conditioning equipment, and traffic),
construction of a "room within a room" is
relatively simple.   There should be at least
a four inch separation between the test room
and the surrounding walls.   The walls of the
room must be made of fairly dense material
(3/4" plywood is a good example), and the
wall separating the test and control rooms
should be structured using a staggered stud
technique.   Double doors of the solid-core
type should be used between the two rooms,
and the window should be a double panel and
heavily glazed (not set tight against the
wood).   Liberal use of carpet and acoustical
tile will reduce reverberation, but will not
contribute significantly to sound attentua-
tion.   Be certain that all openings (electrical, jack panels, etc.) are carefully sealed.
The best made room is of little value if
there is a hole in it.   Proper ventilation

can be accomplished by using sound-absorbing material with several 90° bends leading to and away from the rooms. Fluctuations in sound level from extraneous noise will not significantly affect test results. The acid test for an adequate room is the ability to obtain unoccluded bone conduction thresholds at 0dB HTL.

If construction is impractical or if one has the capital, selection of a manufactured room requires more consideration than ordering it according to exterior dimensions. Be certain that lighting, ventilation, electrical outlets, and jack panels are more than adequate. It is very poor economy to invest in an elaborate and expensive room which becomes too warm, is difficult to see into, and is limited in the number of equipment modalities than can be used. Some rooms have doors that are too small to accomodate patients in wheelchairs, and/or the hallway leading to the room is too narrow. Therefore, pay some attention to accomodation of patients. Also, check to be certain that the window is large enough for good visiion and will not be obstructed by the test equipment. Plan the location of speakers (preferably in opposite corners) and of the patient during testing.

Audiometer, etc. An experienced clinician can perform most of the basic audiometric tests using a portable audiometer with a speech circuit and tape recorder input. By using the monitor circuit through an amplifier, sound-field speech tests in quiet can also be performed. A box of noise makers, such as bicycle horns, bells, and crickets, for checking infants will round out a reasonable system for the beginning practitioner. Certainly, if it can be afforded and justified, a more extensive system is recommended.

When selecting an audiometer, stick to basics. Do not purchase on the basis of gadgetry or exotic tests that are seldom done. Look for a two-channel device with a narrow-band masking circuit. If price is a problem, ask about used and reconditioned audiometers. Keep in mind that a back-up unit will be needed when and if the primary unit is out for repair.

A good sound-field system is important, but it does not have to be a factory unit to be sufficient. High quality microphones, amplifiers, and speakers can be purchased in almost any location, and the audiologist will have a better understanding of the system if he installs and calibrates it himself.

Impedance testing equipment has become a standard addition, and the audiologist should have the equipment necessary to provide this service. The new practitioner is advised to ask fellow professionals about the type of equipment that is most appropriate and serviceable in the area. The clinician seldom needs a recorder to classify tympanograms, and many of the newer portable devices have enough features for the purposes of private practice.

Depending upon the type of practice and its success, the audiologist can consider purchase or lease of a Bekesy-type audiometer, ENG equipment, sound level meter, and hearing aid analyzer. He should keep in mind that neither extensiveness nor expensiveness of equipment is the key to successful practice. Rather, it is volume of work and efficiency of effort, and these goals can be reached without lining the walls with equipment.

Supplies and Office Equipment. Aside from the usual requirements of pens, pencils, carbon, typing paper, paper clips, and rubber bands, the audiologist has some special needs in terms of forms used in practice. If audiologists spent half as much time and money designing intake audiometric and ENG forms as they do designing business cards and stationery, they would all be much better prepared for private practice. The intake form (Fig. 1) should identify the patient referral source, financial obligation, and problem. More than this is seldom necessary since the practitioner can always ask additional questions during and after the examination.

The audiometric evaluation form (Fig. 2) should be easy to interpret and have a sufficient test summary which includes all basic tests (SRT, discrimination, impedance, tone decay, recruitment, etc.). A division of left and right audiograms is strongly recommended. A "two-eared" form is easier to interpret and use for follow-up testing. Lots of space should be available on the audiogram for comments, and this comment space can provide for sufficient interpretation so as to reduce the amount of report writing to referral sources.

Initially, the practitioner is advised to order small quantities of almost everything, especially printed items such as business cards, stationery, and any forms which give names, addresses, and telephone numbers. Too often, such items become obsolete long before the supplies have been used up. Economy of numbers in the formative stage of practice is better than a small savings on larger quantities, which become useless due to change.

Before buying or leasing any office equipment, ask how much it is really needed to provide the services. Do not yield to sales pitch flattery which suggests that success is measured by ownership of a type or variety of machine. Nor is the argument of great tax savings necessarily valid. To pay taxes one must first have income, and if overhead is too high, deductions become a drain on spendable income. If the device seems to be a reasonable acquisition for the practice, request the use of it on a trial rental, or short-term lease. Check into the serviceability of the equipment and the service record of the agent. The most efficient equipment is valueless if there is very much down time.

In addition to furniture items (file cabinets, desks, chairs, lamps, etc.), basic office equipment should include a typewriter, (standard electric), adding machine or print calculator, and dictation equipment. Many practitioners prefer to write out letters, reports, and notes, but that process is inefficient. It is better to learn to use dictation equipment, which saves time and money.

<u>Personnel</u>. Usually, the beginning practitioner has no assistance, but as the practice grows, so does the need for personnel. The search for assistants should be methodical. One should not "just ask around," thus ending up with someone else's problem. Advertise and interview. Use an interview form (Fig. 3) and schedule time to talk with prospects. Be careful that the advertisement and interview form do not discriminate on the basis of race, sex, age, or handicapping conditions. When selecting an assistant in a receptionist-secretary-bookkeeping position, keep in mind the possibility of training the person to perform some basic technical tasks. A

person who can manage the office and also assist in testing is more valuable and will usually take more interest and pride in working. There are, however, at least two potential problems in opting for technical level help. First, if the person assumes too much responsibility, he may try to diagnose the disorder and/or advise the patient. This presents ethical and legal problems, especially in forensic audiology. Second, the person once trained may leave and become competition.

<u>Referral</u> <u>Sources</u> <u>and</u> <u>Bonds</u>. Whether or not one agrees with current prohibitions on advertising, the private audiologist is severely restricted in terms of notifying potential referral sources and the public at large about his services. Formal announcements and telephone listings are inadequate to develop business. The practitioner must compensate by arranging for personal meetings with physicians. In addition to business cards, the audiologist should also have copies of test forms and fee schedules available. Pads of prescription forms with easy-to-follow directions to the office are another device for encouraging referrals. When a referral is received as the result of a contact or notice, the practitioner should respond promptly and express his appreciation.

The open house is a time-honored device of physicians for attracting business by getting aquainted with the professional neighborhood. The practitioner should delay having this function until he has made some aquaintances to assist him in compiling a list of individuals to invite. He should schedule around peak activity times of those he especially wants to come, and he should have friends at the function.

Although formal announcements do not usually yield a large return in referrals, they are useful in getting information about which physicians and agencies are interested in audiology services. Some economy of money and effort will accrue to selective mailing to potential referral sources in the immediate geographic area and to medical specialties that are traditional users of audiometric services (ENT, pediatrics, and neurology).

An acceptable method of advertising is through good work in civic clubs and organizations. The audiologist would do well to select a group in which he has an interest and where medicine and other professions are represented. A speech and hearing group may satisfy certain internal needs for communication with peers, but it does very little for business. Being known as an available speaker for civic groups is another excellent vehicle for informing the public and increasing referrals.

Maintaining a Private Practice. After the decision has been made to begin a practice and the doors are open, how does one keep them open? There is no simple answer or formula that assures success, but there are three principal attitudes which, if adopted, will certainly contribute to growth of the practice. These attitudes are:

1.   Developing clinician-patient relationships.

2.   Becoming a more efficient technician.

3.   Conducting the practice as a business.

Clinician-Patient Relationships. Opportunities for learning the concepts of clinician-patient relationships are limited in the training-center clinic setting. Scheduling problems, changing instructors, charity cases, and semester deadlines all contribute to focusing most of the student's energy on grades, hours, and quantity, and there is not much time available for listening to unrelated or even to related problems of the person the student sees. Further, there is no real contract bond between the audiology student and the patient, whereas, in a private setting, that contract does indeed exist. The patient pays directly for the service and he must be satisfied that the audiologist has his interests foremost at all times.

This interest should be demonstrated from the first contact through the receptionist when the patient makes an appointment, when the patient arrives to fill out pre-examination forms, and when the audiologist greets the patient at the door or in the test room. Speak warmly and smile. Introduce yourself, tell the patient who and what you are and what you are going to do.

When testing is completed, explain the results to the patient and, where indicated, to the family. Do not use technical terms unnecessarily. Go over the "graph of hearing" (audiogram) showing normal hearing (0dB), low and high pitch portions (frequency), and loudness lines (dB HTL). Explain how the patient hears with headphones (air conduction) compared with the vibrator (bone conduction). Verbally or by using a graph explain what part of the hearing mechanism is affected and how.

When a hearing aid is indicated, say so and explain the steps involved in selecting aids. Methods of delivering aids vary widely, so it is difficult to prescribe a system that will work for everyone. However, many audiologists in private practice subscribe to a temporary fitting-brief trial-final fitting approach. Regardless of the system used, it is important to impart to the patient that, as a professional, you are seeking optimum hearing for him. Discussing total cost with a patient who probably will need binaural fitting can be a difficult situation. Remind him that the decision to purchase the aids is ultimately his. Advise the patient that you are available by telephone during the trial period, and that if he has difficulty, he should call.

When the patient returns for the final hearing aid evaluation, take time to determine how he has been doing. This pre-evaluation discussion is helpful for creating a bond with him as well as providing valuable information before formal testing begins. After testing, go over the results in terms of the relative benefit of improved percentage of understanding by comparing unaided and aided discrimination scores.

If the impairment is not amenable to amplification, counsel the patient and his family about the impact of the loss and what should be done or eliminated to provide a good communication environment (this counseling applies equally to the aided patient). If hearing conservation is indicated, discuss the use of ear defenders and the avoidance of noise, both in employment and recreation.

Where medical treatment is being considered to improve hearing or for basic health reasons, the audiologist must refrain from expressing judgements which fall within the realm of the physician. The audiologist must have some prior understanding with the referring physician as to how much information can be revealed without compromising the physician's relationship with his patient. This brings up the painful question as to when, between the physician and the audiologist, the audiologist takes over the patient or becomes the primary provider of services. While audiologists think of themselves as independent practitioners when it comes to amplification, the reality of competition for the health dollar may cause the physician to have a different opinion. It behooves the audiologist to know how the physician feels about audiology services and to act accordingly.

Technical Efficiency. All the foregoing advice about the time required to establish clinician-patient bonds not withstanding, the audiologist cannot afford to waste time during the technical evaluation of the patient. He should get started with testing without delay. Except perhaps for infants, there is little justification for getting into a detailed discussion of the patient's problems before testing. Even in the case of infants, it is better to test first, before child and parent become restive, than it is to engage in lengthy case history taking. The intake form should have sufficient information to provide the audiologist with direction as to how or where testing should proceed.

Keep test instruction short and simple. Most patients will have no difficulty with hand-raising directions, but the more information one gives, the greater the probability of confusion. The audiologist can always reinstruct if a problem occurs. Reduce trips between test and control room. All tests that can be given by air conduction should be completed before bone conduction is performed. These tests include air-conducted

thresholds, SRT's, discrimination, tone
decay, comfort level, recruitment, etc.

Business Practices. Appointments on a desk
pad, accounts in a stenographer's notebook,
and receipts in a shoe box will not do.
Purchase a daily log book and keep appointments in pencil. Ask the patient for a phone
number where he can be reached. (The audiologist will also occasionally have to cancel
and rearrange appointments.) In addition to
patient files for audiograms and reports,
keep small cards with patient-identifying
information on the front and services performed, by date and fees charged on the back.
This smaller system allows the audiologist to
review quickly what he has done and when he
has done it. Keep all files alphabetically
and by year.

As yet, there are no accounting systems
available which have been designed specifically for audiologists, but those systems
designed for dentists are sufficiently similar to be adapted for audiology. The use of
an accounting firm with experience in setting
up and auditing books for dentists and physicians is recommended. Few, if any, audiologists comprehend or can keep up with state
and federal requirements for accounting and
paying the several taxes (income, property,
employment security, etc.) which exist as a
part of the business world.

The Audiologist and the Otologist

Audiology's development has been called
a product of the combining of the field of
speech pathology and the medical specialty of
otology. The contributions of psychology,
acoustics, electronics, and deaf education
have often been overlooked in terms of both
education and practice. Vast improvements in

the field of medical electronics as well as a greater public awareness of the needs of the handicapped have created a phenomenal growth in training and research programs in the field of audiology. This growth has moved at such an accelerating pace that many training programs have found themselves in the position of producing "audiologists" who move immediately to another academic location to establish another training program which in turn produces more "audiologists," etc., etc., etc.

The great variety of specialized electronic and acoustic apparatus has caused many educators in the field to oversimplify the responsibilities of the clinical audiologist. Obviously, if the only function of the audiologist ever observed by those in the field of medicine is the obtaining of pure tone air and bone thresholds to confirm the clinical observations of the otologist, then it would certainly be difficult to convince a physician in the specialty of otology that he should consider including in his practice someone who has nine or ten years of college training and certain affiliations and certificates attesting to his clinical competence in audiology.

Let us now suppose a situation in which an otologist is to decide whether audiology services should be made available to his patients, and, if so, what kind. One obvious and seemingly inexpensive choice would be for the physician to purchase directly from an audiometer manufacturer equipment that would enable him, or one of his employees, to administer certain essential tests to determine and/or confirm the desirability of surgical and/or medical procedures. Since the performance of pure tone air, bone tests, and certain speech tests appears to be relatively simple, the physician may order one of many instruments that can perform these functions.

After entering private practice, I began a survey of equipment and services available in physicians' offices, and found that there were many standard clinical audiometers as well as those having more extensive and expensive automatic features. Reported investments in this equipment, exclusive of the audiometric test suite, ranged from approximately $1,500 to $7,000. In addition, much of this equipment was gathering dust for one of at least three reasons: (1) The otologist soon found that he did not have sufficient time to devote to performing a battery of tests. (2) Without someone to provide appropriate education and supervision of the "technician," the instrumentation and/or the test conditions tended to over-whelm many of those selected within the office to perform the requested tests. (3) "Strange" readings appeared with regard to comparison of air and bone conduction thresh-olds, thus necessitating continued and frus-trating service calls from the audiometer representative.

Let us now consider an audiologist who is thinking of establishing a clinic program either with or independent of an otologist. Let us further assume that his training has been similar to that of an applicant inter-viewed recently regarding the possibility of going into private practice. The clinic environment from which he has recently grad-uated is an affluent one. Numerous double-walled steel test rooms and single- or double-walled control enclosures have been available for his use. He has had available a sophisticated dual channel clinical audio-meter with short increment sensitivity index (SISI) and warble tone adaptors, not to mention such things as narrow-band masking, intercom override button, and a host of glowing lights, sliding switches, and gleaming dials. He has also had a Bekesy-type audiometer as well as at least one rack of ultraspecialized equipment, which he has been asked to use for data gathering for someone's experiment. Let us assume also that the essential medical history has been obtained by a receptionist, and that after one or more hours of testing, he has retired to an office or cubicle in order to compose a detailed report of test results, patient behavior, and guarded conclusions, while avoiding direct diagnostic terminology. He is often ignorant of the fees charged to the various clients for the various services, and is almost never required to discuss them with the family. If a hearing aid is a possibility, he usually recommends that the patient return to the clinic at some future date for an evaluation. If auditory training, lipreading, or counseling for deaf education appear to be indicated, he makes the recommendation and suggests referral to some other division within the clinic for completion of this nonaudiometric service.

In the course of the conversation with this applicant I asked him to provide me with a list of the minimum equipment required for a comprehensive practice, the tests to be performed, the services to be offered, the charges to be made for services, the proposed location of the practice, and the number of patients he expected to see each day. After a careful analysis of his list, I concluded that for each day of operation of his office in private practice he would increase his indebtedness approximately $125.

The point is not that audiologists are incompetent, but rather that they have, through a process of educational expediency, assumed the role of technician and have been inadequately informed regarding private practice in audiology. They have, as it were, been caught in an environment which may view the patient as an object of study for training rather than as an individual they are being trained to serve.

From these two examples of otology and audiology planning services, some meaningful conclusions about positive relationships which can and do exist between otology and audiology can be drawn. Another alternative is the inclusion, assistance, or referral to audiology.

The clinical or rehabilitation audiologist does, of course, concern himself with the measurement and function of the auditory system. He must be adequately equipped, trained, and interested in the patient so that he may provide the otologist, on request, confirmatory evidence of the advisability of medical and/or surgical treatment. If both otology and audiology assume these aspects of audiology as the only, or even as the primary, role of audiology, then the audiologist is certainly doomed to replacement by automation and the audiometric technician.

The enlightened and concerned otologist and, I hope, the enlightened and concerned audiologist will recognize that once medicine and surgery have reached their limits of hearing restoration, the patient should now return to the audiologist for auditory rehabilitation.

The first question concerns amplification or hearing aids. I do not wish to engage in questions of medical ethics, rights, or responsibilities for the direct referral from the otologist to the hearing aid dealer.   I have often found myself more at odds with my colleagues in audiology, regarding their bad habits in the fitting of hearing aids, than I have with the otologists who may insist that direct referrals to an "honest" or "reputable" hearing aid dealer do as much good as referral to an audiological clinic. The student clinician in training in audiology cannot possibly know enough about the dealers, the various instruments in the clinic, the dealer's service record and reputation, the guarantees of the instruments, or even whether the individual who receives the instrument can be expected to receive any further service when he goes home. The private practitioner, however, usually is highly selective in terms of dealers and instruments. He is usually personally acquainted with the dealer and has carefully discussed each instrument chosen to be included in his clinic armament.   In addition, he will usually impose certain rules of conduct upon the dealer with regard to patients referred to him by the audiologist, e.g., an extended free trial period at no cost to the patient. The private practitioner expects a report from the dealer concerning follow-up contacts with the patient, and expects the patient to return to his office for a follow-up consultation. He includes as a part of the evaluation process, time set aside for counseling with the patient concerning problems that may arise with the instrument or its adjustment. He also counsels with the patient's family regarding the effect of the hearing loss and the use of amplification.

In the case of the pediatric patient, the private audiologist will proceed with caution in terms of the use of amplification and will require the cooperative involvement of the otologist in determining stages of amplification. The audiologist counsels with the parents regarding the impact of the hearing loss on the child; he also discusses the feelings of the parents, assists in designing language and speech training programs at home (if the audiologist is fortunate enough to have the time and/or staff to pursue a separate therapy program), and advises parents about various educational programs available. The audiologist exercises similar caution in the use of amplification with the older patient and in counseling with the relatives of the patient.

The audiologist should have available, or be able to refer to, sources of additional education of the deaf and hard-of-hearing child as well as lipreading and auditory training classes for the adult.

The audiologist may also operate in the area of industrial audiometry or hearing conservation in determining damage-risk criteria, preemployment audiograms for baseline, referral to an otologist for individuals found to have hearing loss, the selection and education of workers in the use of ear defenders, etc.

The conditions under which audiologists operate as private practitioners vary considerably from location to location. It is not always the extensiveness of the equipment that determines the quality of the program. One of the finest audiology programs I have seen, in terms of quality testing, service, and management of hearing disorders, had a total investment of less than $1,000 and included the capacity for the testing of hearing aids in a controlled sound environment. The other extreme exists where $30,000 worth of equipment was being used mainly to provide air and bone tests, while those individuals who could not be helped medically or surgically were referred out of the clinic directly to the hearing aid center.

The audiologist also serves as a consultant in the selection of appropriate equipment for the services to be rendered. Quiet environments are a must for the performance of most tests, but this does not necessarily mean the expense of portable sound-treated rooms. Certainly, the otologist is interested in his ability to pursue suspected retrocochlear involvement, but this does not necessarily require the expense of SISI and/or Bekesy units. Early diagnostic information concerning the extent of hearing loss in infants is of major concern to both audiologists and otologists, but this does not necessarily require the expense of evoked response audiometry or galvanic skin response (GSR) audiometry. If the otologist elects to provide his own diagnostic information in full or in part, he would be well advised to discuss his problems and needs with persons other than the research audiologist or the salesman handling the equipment.

The maintenance of equipment also merits consideration. Valid air, bone, and other types of audiometric information may not be obtained except under certain quiet, sound-field conditions because of the masking effect of bandwidths of noise on the frequencies in question. For example, sufficient ambient noise may exist in these lower frequencies in a room where an air and bone pure tone test is being made to show a hearing loss where none actually exists. The use of specially constructed muffs will assist in the validation of the air conduction tests, but spurious readings by bone conduction remain unaffected. Tolerances in the calibration of audiometric equipment are rather large (plus or minus 3 to 4 dB) and continued use, jarring, dropping, or overdriving either headphones or bone oscillators can appreciably alter the calibration of the equipment. Without frequent routine checks of the calibration of this equipment, neither the audiologist nor the otologist can place much confidence in the results of the findings. The fact that the machine may be occasionally returned to the factory for recalibration does not ensure that it will remain in calibration until it reaches the physician's office.

Electronystagmography, in clinics where it exists, is considered by both otologists and audiologists to be within the realm of audiology as an additional diagnostic test, in which data are charted, analyzed, and forwarded to the otologist for interpretation. It is a rather expensive procedure, in terms of both equipment and time, but where it is used, physicians seem convinced of its desirability.

What are some of the other otology-audiology arrangements that exist in the United States? We have already discussed briefly the technician arrangement in which the otologist employs someone with less than the education and training recommended by the American Speech and Hearing Association on a salaried basis. Usually there are no additional charges for the audiometrics performed by this individual, and these charges are included and/or absorbed in the regular examination fees or the post-surgical fees of the physician.

Another common arrangement is the employment, by the otologist and/or otologic group, of an audiologist who meets ASHA standards. The equipment is usually purchased by the physician or medical group, and the audiologist works on a salary or a salary plus a percentage of the gross income of the audiology clinic. This audiologist usually sees only those persons referred to him by the physician or the group by which he is employed. Two problems observed in this arrangement are that the audiologist has a tendency to become "technician" oriented, and that there is often a reluctance on the part of other physicians, who may feel the need of audiometric information, to refer patients to the group.

A similar arrangement is one in which a supervising or consulting audiologist is employed by the physician or group, with the equipment still purchased by the physicians. The supervising audiologist is responsible for the provision of services to patients referred by the otologist. He may employ one or more additional audiologists and/or audiometric technicians to assist in the collection of routine audiometric information, but he retains the responsibility for the quality of the work performed, the provision of counseling services when required, and the maintenance of the equipment.

Professional corporation arrangements have also been noted among otologists and audiologists. This is not greatly dissimilar to the employee or employee-consultant status, except that the audiologist may benefit from a greater "draw" as well as improved retirement and tax benefits.

Still another arrangement is the associate status, in which the audiologist and otologist share office space. There also may be some sharing of equipment costs and office staff for purposes of billing. There is cross-referral, but the associate audiologist accepts referrals from other physicians, and refers to the ear, nose, and throat (ENT) specialist only with the permission of the referring physician.

Finally, there is the independent audiologist who offers his clinic facility as a source of referral from physicians for diagnostic work-ups, amplification, and other forms of auditory rehabilitation.

In terms of the relative salaries and costs of audiology and audiologists, the physician accustomed to employing nurses, LPN's, receptionists, technicians, etc., may feel that the money demanded by the audiologist for his services is unreasonable. The otologist should keep in mind that only a portion of his income is derived from the office practice, while a much larger portion of his income may come from surgery. The audiologist, on the other hand, has no operating room; however, the dispensing of hearing aids may serve the audiologist in much the same way as surgery does the otologist.

The office overhead costs of the audiologist are seldom less than those of the otologist, and in some instances may be slightly higher. The amount of time normally required for a complete hearing evaluation (assuming no unforeseen difficulties arise) is 45 minutes. In addition, the audiologist must take some time to record his information and to discuss his findings with the patient. This may bring the total time per patient to over one hour. During the time the audiologist is examining one patient, the otologist may see up to ten. This comparison is not meant to suggest that the otologist does not spend enough time with his patient, but simply to point out that the time requirements of the examinations are not comparable. (The audiologist in private practice sometimes also suffers from existing scales of costs of services presented by community or university clinics that benefit from considerable local, state, and federal support.)

Some examples of salaries follow:

Example A: A certified master's degree level audiologist is employed at a guaranteed salary of $12,000 plus a percentage of the gross income of the audiological business, which increases with time (perhaps 2% to 3% per year, up to 10% of this gross income). The equipment is supplied by the otologist.

Example B: The corporate members (of which the master's degree level certified audiologist is one) share in the proceeds at a minimum of $1,500 per month, plus a percentage of the income of the individual's portion over that amount, plus a contribution to retirement. Equipment is owned by the corporation.

Example C: The doctoral level audiologist is an employee of a medical group of four otologists. He supervises the program, which employs five additional persons. He has a base salary of $25,000, plus 9% of the gross income, plus available time for outside consultation and teaching.

Example D: A doctoral level audiologist supervises the program for a medical group of six otologists on a consulting basis at $200 per day. He has permission to examine individuals referred directly to him and to bill separately for the patients. All other referrals are from the medical group, and this income is returned to the audiology center for its operation. That center employs four other persons.

Example E: The associate audiologist at the doctoral level shares the offices of

the otologist and purchases and/or
leases his own equipment. He sets the
charges and does his billing through the
physician's facility, paying a comparable overhead rate for the use of the
space and billing costs. The associate
accepts outside referrals from other
physicians, including other ear, nose,
and throat specialists.

Example F: A doctoral level, supervising consultant in audiology is responsible for meeting the audiologic needs
of two otologists during the time the
otologists are in the office. This
requires approximately 15 hours per week
of the audiologist's time, and utilizes
auxillary personnel as well. The equipment is supplied by the physician.

Example G: The totally independent
audiologist (very rare indeed) has his
income determined solely by his ability
to attract sufficient referrals, charge
appropriate fees, etc. No figures are
available on his exact income.

The reported cost for services in all
instances was given as a minimum base cost of
$25 per hour based on charges from private
practice clinics in various states. However,
these are the larger clinics, which are able
to employ auxillary personnel and to operate
with large otological groups, and therefore
remain quite busy.

For services limited to pure tone air
and bone testing, which the reporting clinics
consider appropriate only as preemployment
audiograms, the charge is $10.

For hearing evaluations, which include
pure tone air and bone, speech reception
thresholds, discrimination scores, and mea-

surements of communicative ability in the sound field, the charge is $20 to $25.

For hearing aid evaluations, which include the measurement of speech reception thresholds, discrimination scores, comfortable loudness, tolerance, etc. on three to four instruments considered to be most suitable for the patient, the charge is $35 to $40.

For earmolds in the clinic the charge is $10 to $15.

For initial pediatric evaluation and interview the charge is $25.

For follow-up pediatric tests and special tests such as SISI, Bekesy, etc., the charges are $5 per 15 minutes.

Therapy and counseling are provided at the rate of $20 per 45 minute session, or portion thereof.

All of the foregoing is not to imply that otology is remiss in its efforts to provide the best of care for and management of patients with hearing disorders. The quarrel, if any, is usually with those audiologists who have often failed to show leadership and practical application of their training to the otologists. For those patients for whom medicine has reached its limits in terms of restoration of hearing and a communicative problem still exists, the audiologist should seek to educate the otologist through, for example, efficient and prompt reporting as well as follow-up and concern. Perhaps with assistance, urgence, patience, and professional interaction from otology, audiology may yet take its place not under and not in place of but alongside the field of otology in the management of hearing disorders.

APPENDIX

CHAPTER VIII

AUDIOLOGY LABORATORY

Patient's   Child
Full   Miss
Name   Mrs.
                   Mr. _____
                             Last   First   Middle

Male _____ Female _____   Age: _____

Birthdate: _____
              Month   Day   Year

Address: _____   Phone: _____
           Street & Number   City & State   Zip Code

Name of person who will pay account: _____

Address of above person: _____   Phone: _____

232

Employment of responsible person: _____ Phone: _____

Who referred you to doctor: _____

Insurance Company: _____

Medicare No.: _____ Welfare No.: _____

Type of trouble you are having: _____

_____

Date: _____
        Current Date

FIGURE 1

FROM: Audiology Laboratory
1201 Classen Drive
Oklahoma City, OK 73103

Phone: 235-3371

TO: _____

ADDRESS: _____

CITY: _____

Date: _____

The above named patient was seen in this office for an audiometric evaluation at the request of

Dr. _____, Otolaryngologist, for diagnostic purposes and not to

determine type of hearing aid.

Procedure	Left Ear	Right Ear	Binaurally	Charge
Pure Tone Air and Bone				$
Speech Discrimination				
Speech Reception Thresholds				
Tone Decay				
Impedance				

234

Recruitment _____ ___ ___ ___

Diplacusis _____ ___ ___ ___

Weber _____ ___ ___ ___

Bing _____ ___ ___ ___

Stenger ___ ___

TOTAL BALANCE DUE $ _____

Less any payments - _____

Any Balance DUE $ _____

Impression: _____

Dr. Roy C. Rowland, Jr., Ph.D., is approved for the above named services. ID No. **73**-0786878.

_____

Roy C. Rowland, Jr., Ph.D.

Audiologist

FIGURE 2

EMPLOYMENT APPLICATION

Date: _____

SS#: _____

Name: _____ Brith Date: _____ Age: ____
(Print)   First   Middle   Last

Address: _____ Phone: _____

Birth Place: _____ Position applying for: _____

Physical Defects: _____

Marital Status: (check one) □ Single □ Married □ Separated □ Divorced □ Widowed

Number of Dependents: _____ Spouse's Name: _____

Spouse's Employment: _____ Years employed: _____
                          Name

Address: _____ Phone: _____
         Street & Number   City & State   Zip Code

Parents name: _____ Phone: _____

Address: _____
         Street & Number   City & State   Zip Code

EDUCATION

Check the last completed:

Grades below high school	□ 1	□ 2	□ 3	□ 4	□ 5	□ 6	□ 7	□ 8
High school	□ 9	□ 10	□ 11	□ 12				
College	□ 1	□ 2	□ 3	□ 4	□ 5			

High School Attended: _____

College Attended: _____

Business or Technical School Attended: _____

TECHNICAL SKILLS

Typing WPM _____ Dictaphone _____ Adding Machine _____

Posting Machine _____ Shorthand _____

Describe other types of machines about which you are knowledgeable: _____

FIGURE 3

237

AUDIOLOGY LABORATORY

===

Roy C. Rowland, Jr. Ph.D.
1201 Classen Drive
Oklahoma City, Oklahoma 73103

Please find enclosed one statement. This statement is the ATTENDING PHYSICIAN'S STATE-MENT, or ITEMIZED STATEMENT, needed to file an insurance claim. Attach this statement to your claim form and send it to your insurance company for payment of your benefit. This is the only itemized statement that you will receive.

We have no contract with insurers or Medi-care. Our only contract is with you, as your private audiologist. We will therefore look only to you for payment.

If this office can be of further service to you, please don't hesitate to call upon us.

Accts. Secretary

FIGURE 4

FRONT OF CARD

Name: _____ BD: _____

Address: _____ Age: _____

                                       Phone: _____

Resp. Party: _____

Ref. Dr.: _____ Bill: _____

Ins./Ma.: _____

Complaint: _____

Recheck after: RX _____ 6 Mo. _____ 1 Yr. _____ HA. Fitting _____

              Other _____

COMMENTS:

239

BACK OF CARD

DATE	CHARGE	BAL.

FIGURE 5

CHAPTER IX

ELECTRONYSTAGMOGRAPHY:
ITS ROLE AND FUNCTION IN
AUDIOLOGICAL PRIVATE PRACTICE

Darrell L. Teter, Ph.D.

Introduction and Overview of Chapter

A decision had to be made concerning
this chapter, as to whether the contents
would be directed toward discussing the
physiology of nystagmus and the interpretation of the test battery, or whether this
book's intended readers would benefit more
from a discussion centered on the practical
and professional questions involving the
audiologist providing ENG in a private practice setting.

Since many texts contain sections on ENG
and some are devoted entirely to ENG, any
contribution made by this material, had it
been directed towards physiology and the
interpretation of ENG, would not have been
significant. However, there is no text that
deals with the philosophies, equipment, and
financial concerns of the audiologist providing ENG testing. This chapter will thus be
directed toward those areas. It will not
discuss in detail the ENG test battery or its
full interpretation. Rather, it will discuss
philosophies, economics, equipment, space,
financial considerations, and, finally, the
manner in which the audiologist can best
report the ENG findings.

It is the author's wish that the information provided within this chapter assist

all of those audiologists interested in
providing ENG within the framework of a
private audiological practice.

A Brief History of ENG

Although the technique of ENG has been
available for 30 years, it has only been in
the last five to seven years that the technique has achieved widespread use and acceptance. This delay in acceptance has been, in
part, due to the normal resistance of the
professionals involved to accept electro-
physiological measurements and techniques
requiring amplifiers and recorders. In part,
the reluctance has also been due to some of
the difficulties encountered with early
amplifiers and recorders.

Early in its infancy, ENG was recommended over the clinical use of ice water
calorics because ENG was said to provide an
objective, repeatable, and reliable method of
measuring vestibular function. In reality,
however, the early equipment often did not
control stimulus parameters and thus did not
provide reliable, repeatable measurements.
As a result, ENG techniques were often in
doubt and the technique did not gain rapid
acceptance on the part of physicians and
other clinicians.

The equipment today offers ease of
operation, with highly reliable temperature
and time controls. When performed by the
trained individual (Fig. 1), the results
obtained are accurate, reliable, and repeatable. Unfortunately, not all of the professionals that could benefit from the knowledge
available from ENG are aware of the vast
improvement in equipment and, thus, the vast
improvement in information obtained. Because
of this lag in awareness, ENG has only

recently begun to assume its rightful role in
the practice of medicine and audiology. The
interest in and use of ENG has expanded
rapidly in recent years and will understand-
ably continue to do so. As ENG increases in
use, more knowledge is obtained, and this
perpetuates its own growth and value.

The Purpose of ENG

The overall purpose of ENG is, of
course, to assist in the evaluation of the
"dizzy" patient. More specifically, ENG
serves to provide data to establish whether
dizziness is secondary to a vestibular disorder or if the dizziness is secondary to a
central nervous system disorder. Thus, it
can be said that electronystagmography
assists in localizing the source of dizziness.

The Advantages of ENG

The ENG test battery has several advantages over other methods of evaluating the
vestibular and oculomotor mechanisms of the
dizzy patient. The major advantages are:

1.   ENG allows for the recording and
     measurement of nystagmus behind
     closed eyes. Since most nystagmus
     exists only when the eyes are
     closed, the ENG allows for seeing
     pathological nystagmus missed by
     other methods.

2.   ENG provides a reliable, permanent,
     and objective record of the pa-
     tient's response to movement and to
     caloric stimulation.

3. The ENG test battery is a valuable asset in evaluating medical therapy, pre- and post-surgery changes, and long-term changes in vestibular function; it is virtually a necessity in medical-legal evaluations, since only the ENG test battery provides a repeatable, controlled, reliable, and objective method of measuring changes in a patient's vestibular system.

Professional Considerations Concerning ENG

ENG testing has been caught for many years in a controversy involving domain. The test battery is done to provide the physician with information to assist him or her in making a diagnosis involving the dizzy patient. With the localizing information provided by ENG, such a diagnosis is often possible. In no way does the ENG test or its interpretation make a diagnosis. The data obtained allow the physician to make that diagnosis. Since the physician has ordered the test and uses the data, the ENG equipment has historically been owned by the physician or physician groups and the testing has been done by technicians.

As the demands for testing increased and the equipment and test battery became more complex, many professionals felt that technicians could not always handle the complexities and the demands of ENG. The increased cost of the equipment made it more difficult for solo practitioners in medicine to purchase the ENG equipment and ENG test facilities have, of late, been established in hospitals or in private audiological practices, often independent of a physician in practice.

The combination of increased demands, increased complexity, increased costs, and establishment of private practice audiological facilities to provide ENG testing, all brought to the forefront questions as to the exact role of the audiologist in evaluating the dizzy patient. That question (or questions) cannot be answered in total here; however, some very important considerations based on the author's experience may assist the reader in making some conclusions concerning the physician-audiologist relationship in providing ENG's and the role of ENG's in a private audiological practice.

The ENG test battery is a demanding and structured one, if it is to be well done. Knowledge of instrumentation and vestibular anatomy and physiology, and the ability to observe and relate the patient's history to observations as well as indications for testing, have all contributed to bringing the audiologist, rather than the technician, into ENG testing. Some audiologists feel that ENG testing places them in the role of a technician, and for that reason will not perform ENG's. I believe that these individuals simply have not had enough experience with electronystagmography and its interpretation, or they would not consider the audiologist's role a technician's role.

At the other end of the continuum, in terms of philosophy, are the audiologists who realize the power of a good ENG test battery and its contribution to making a diagnosis concerning the dizzy patient. These individuals know the demands of providing good ENG data; they realize the contributions that ENG's done by audiologists can make in patient care, as well as the benefit to themselves professionally and financially. They also add one more dimension to the audiologist's role in providing good, comprehensive hearing health care.

The audiologist providing ENG testing soon learns, however, that there are pluses as well as minuses assoicated with ENG testing. Some of the most obvious will be discussed briefly in the sections that follow.

Cost

The equipment necessary to provide ENG varies in total cost depending upon the quality and capabilities of the equipment purchased. A quality single channel ENG unit with an irrigator ranges in cost from $3,000 to $4,000. Obviously, equipment costs of this nature dictate sufficient use of the equipment to justify the capital expenditure. The addition of a suitable testing table or chair, when one is not immediately available, will add an additional $600 to $1,200 to the total cost. Special accessories such as digital light bars, optical calibration systems, or optical OPK systems will add another $1,000 to the cost of the equipment. A good quality dual channel ENG unit with all accessories costs approximately $5,000.

In additon to the capital investment necessary to purchase ENG equipment, ENG testing also demands expenditures in terms of time and space. A complete battery of ENG tests requires approximately one and a half hours to two hours. Attempts at reducing this time expenditure almost always reduce the amount of information obtained. The space requirements for ENG must also be included in the expenditure column. An adequate ENG room must be no smaller than 8 x 10 feet and preferrably closer to 12 x 10. The room must contain the ENG equipment and table, as well as a sink and storage space. It is not often that the space allotted for

ENG can also be used for other purposes. Thus, at today's space costs, another monetary consideration must be added when providing ENG testing facilities. The ENG test room should be chosen so that it is isolated from distractions and so that the light level can be controlled.

When totalling the cost of equipment, space, personnel, and time, ENG testing is not an expenditure lightly considered or readily justified for every audiological practice.

Derived Income

The cost to the patient for an ENG test battery varies according to the location of the practice providing the services. The author's experience indicates a price range from $50 to $100 with the most common fees somewhere between $65 and $75. This is for the ENG test battery and its interpretation . Often the total battery of tests includes audiometrics, with additional cost considerations.

When considering equipment costs, ENG space requirements, time requirements, and personnel costs, ENG testing does not always serve as a large revenue producer, unless it is part of an established practice with a large patient load. An audiologist just starting practice, however, may wish to add ENG's to provide more complete services to his or her potential referring sources. Such reasoning has much more merit than adding ENG as a money-maker, since it requires a considerable patient load for a long period of time to offset the capital investments and the time and space investments necessary to provide ENG on a profitable basis.

The audiologist providing good ENG testing will derive many indirect benefits, however. These include a broadening of potential referral sources to include many medical specialties, such as neurology, neurosurgery, and forensic medicine, as well as an opportunity to provide services for individuals who may return to the audiologist's office for additional audiological-related services.

As a service necessary for providing total audiological care, ENG is essential to the overall productivity and performance of a private audiological practice. Without a referral base to provide five to six ENG tests per week, however, the service will not prove to be financially self-supporting. Such monetary facts must be considered along with professional demands before one attempts to provide ENG in a private audiological practice.

Professional Liability

Another consideration for the audiologist providing ENG's is that of any potential professional liability. A few professionals have expressed concern that the actual act of irrigating an ear may expose them to high risk in terms of liability. More than ten years of experience by this author has failed to demonstrate any increased risk secondary to providing ENG's as part of our practice.

It must be remembered that there is a real possibility of creating an infection secondary to irrigating an ear in the instance of a perforated tympanic membrane. If normal precautions are taken to note the presence of a perforation, however, no irrigation should ever by performed on an ear with a perforated tympanic membrane. Should such an error occur, however, the patient should be sent back to the referring source so that the appropriate medical steps can be taken.

In reality, there is no real increase in liability secondary to providing ENG services. There is, of course, increased responsibility to see that perforated ears are not irrigated and that ears are not traumatized with the speculum during irrigation. This responsibility is well within the bounds of the audiologist providing ENG's and should not in itself serve as a deterrent to the audiologist interested in performing ENG's.

The question of how to deal with greatly impacted cerumen in the ear of a patient referred for ENG always is raised. The answer is a simple one: Check the canals before doing anything and if they are impacted, send the patient back to the referring source. Removal of cerumen is the physician's responsibility.

ENG Equipment Considerations

The purchase of ENG equipment requires careful consideration in order to obtain the most dependable and versatile equipment for the money expended. Attempts to utilize recorders and irrigators which are not specifically designed for ENG testing meet with disaster. The major equipment considerations will be discussed in the following sections.

ENG Recorders

The ENG recorder should, of course, be reliable and accurate, as are virtually all of today's commercially available units. In

addition to the obvious demands for accuracy
and reliability, an ENG recorder should have:

1. AC and DC coupling so that eye
    movements may be recorded in rela-
    tion to their true position (DC)
    and, when necessary, by AC coupl-
    ing, in cases where abberent eye
    movements are such that a good
    recording cannot be made. In
    practice, the DC coupling is the
    easiest to calibrate and can be
    used for most subjects. The most
    acceptable time constant for AC
    units is approximately three
    seconds. Quality recorders offer
    either AC or DC coupling simply by
    flipping a switch.

2. Two-speed chart drives on the
    recorder are essential because the
    slower speed can be used for cali-
    bration while the actual test is
    run at a higher speed for improved
    accuracy and recording response.
    The most common and acceptable
    speeds are 5 mm/second and 10
    mm/second. The chart speed during
    recording must be known if the
    nystagmoid movements are to be
    measured using the speed of the
    response as a parameter.

3. Two-channel recording capability is
    most desirable. Often the addi-
    tional expenditure for a dual
    channel recorder forces a decision
    to use a single unit. Experienced
    clinicians who have truly evaluated
    the demands of good ENG recordings
    realize that dual channel capabili-
    ties are essential. The second
    channel will allow the recording of
    vertical nystagmus, which is usu-

ally indicative of CNS involvement, as well as the recording of any vertical movements in the form of muscle potentials, such as eye-blinks, that can quite easily be read as a horizontal nystagmus.

In some ENG recorders, the second channel also can be used as a velocity coupler to record the derived velocity of the horizontal nystagmus recorded on the first channel. The best possible dual channel arrangement allows the second channel to record vertical nystagmus or, by means of switching, to record the derivative of the horizontal nystagmus. The derivative information can be time-saving in many recording situations. Purchasing a second channel or an accessory channel, which is solely a derivative measuring device, is not economically wise.

Irrigation Systems

The ENG test battery revolves around bithermal calorics and thus demands accurate control of water temperature and the amount of water delivered. The irrigation system and its capabilities are vital to good ENG testing (Fig. 1).

Good irrigation systems should provide the following:

1. Adequate capacity for several irrigations without the need to refill the tanks.

2. Temperature control within one-half a degree Centigrade of the required temperatures (7° above and 7° below average body temperature).

3.   Careful timing of the duration of
      the irrigation. In some ENG units,
      the timing of the irrigation is
      controlled by the mechanism within
      the irrigator; in others, the
      timers are in the recording system.
      Either way, it is essential that
      the times be accurate and consis-
      tent. Automatic timers that start
      the irrigation, start and stop the
      recorder, and stop the irrigation
      are essential so that the individ-
      ual doing the testing need not
      bother with all the mechanics of
      the irrigation. Since the criteria
      for measuring caloric responses
      call for at least 20% accuracy, the
      temperature and time controls must
      be within this range of accuracy.

4.   A well-designed irrigation system
      that utilizes heating elements that
      are not exposed to the water and
      thus do not require distilled water
      to avoid mineral deposits.

5.   Temperature indicators that are
      located so as always to be in the
      water, regardless of the water
      level. If they are not, there is a
      danger of delivering overheated
      water.

6.   A warning system to advise when
      water levels are low, to avoid
      overheating and starting an irri-
      gation without sufficient water to
      complete the irrigation.

7.   A pump to provide adequate irriga-
      tion without using gravity and to
      allow water to be recirculated when
      purging the system before irriga-
      tion. This reduces errors, saves

water, and assures adequate water delivery for irrigation.

8. An automatic drain, so that the tanks may be readily emptied for cleaning or for transportation.

9. Some form of indication that tells the tester when the irrigation system is pumping the water. This avoids errors and accidents caused by inadvertantly activating the irrigator.

10. Some form of "abort" button so that at a touch the irrigation and recording can be stopped. This is valuable in cases where the patient becomes ill during an irrigation and it is desirable to immediately stop water delivery and the recorder.

11. A water delivery system that is activated by a two-way foot-operated switch, or a dual action foot switch. When activated by pushing on one side (or on the first activation), the pump is started and purges the system. When activated by pushing the other side (or on the second activation), the pump is started under control of the timers, which time the irrigation and start the recorder either after the irrigation or simultaneously with the irrigation.

It should be readily apparent that the caloric irrigator is an essential part of the entire ENG test system and as such must be chosen as carefully as the recorder. A poorly designed irrigation system is a source of trouble.

Air vs. Water

At this point in our discussion, it is essential to mention the use of air rather than water as the caloric stimulus. The opponents of water cite two problems inherent in its use: (1) the mess and inconvenience in filling the tanks, irrigating the ear, and then disposing of the water after the irrigation; and (2) the fact that an ear with a perforated drum cannot be irrigated using water, due to the risk of infection. Conversely, the proponents of air note that their system involves no mess in using air as a stimulus, and that air can be used in an ear with a tympanic membrane perforation without fear of infection.

Careful consideration of some of the realities of ENG should provide some assistance for those attempting to decide whether an air or water system should be purchased. Consider, for example, how often it would be informative to do an ENG on a perforated ear. Regardless of the method used the stimulus delivered to that ear would be greater than that to the other vestibular mechanism, and one could determine only if the labyrinth on the perforated side is working or not. No comparison could be made between the vestibular mechanisms since the stimulus delivered would not be equal. The use of air in such a circumstance is complicated by the fact that any moisture in the canal will alter the temperature of the stimulus and offset expected responses.

In reality, the need for irrigation of perforated ears is not very great. Also, experienced clincians do not find the use of water to be an inconvenience or a mess. The advantages of water include many years of data concerning the expected responses and the fact that water has proven to be much more dependable and repeatable in terms of response parameters. Air has not given most clinicians repeatable results, even with the longer stimulus parameters and increased temperatures required by air. I much prefer water over air and find no real advantage to air caloric systems.

Chair and/or Exam Table Requirements

The choice of a proper exam chair or table is an important one in assembling adequate ENG equipment. The chair must be stable and comfortable and must recline so that the patient can be supine. In addition to reclining to a supine position, the arms of the chair should be moveable so that the patient can be placed in Hallpike positions.

Any table used for ENG needs to be of stable width (34 to 36 inches), padded so as to be comfortable, and adjustable from a sitting to a supine position (Fig. 2). The cost of an ENG examining table or chair varies from $600 to $1,200.

Pretest Instructions

The wise audiologist will provide the ENG patient with a very specific list of pretest instructions. These instructions have two purposes: (1) to guarantee that no medications or stimulants have been taken that will alter the vestibular system, and (2) to keep the stomach empty in case the calorics induce vomiting.

The pretest instructions used in the author's office are included in the Appendix (Fig. 3). Every practice will want to develop its own pretest instructions and explanations.

Pretest History

The complexity of the pretest history done in the audiologist's office depends, in part, upon the referring source. Often the referring source will do a complete history as part of the medical evaluaton. Many times a prearranged history form will be used and filled out at the time of testing to be sent with the test results. That form should be designed by the referral source and the professionals providing services. Included on any history form should be the following:

1. patient's description of symptoms,

2. onset and circumstances surrounding onset,

3. a definite description of any positional vertigo.

This information is of value in providing adequate testing and in interpreting results. For example, all ENG tests should include an effort to duplicate any head or body position that produces vertigo. Considerable information can also be obtained by asking the patient to describe his clinical symptoms in relation to the sensation induced by the calorics; thus, the necessity of a history to elicit positional complaints and the importance of reporting the subjective resonse to the calorics.

Factors to Consider When
Obtaining the History

1. Patient's own description of complaint
    (Try to get the patient to describe
    dizziness without using terms such as
    "dizzy" or "vertigo.")

2. Approximate date of onset
    a. Was there illness or accident at
        that time?
    b. Has it worsened, improved, or
        stayed the same?
    c. Are symptoms episodic, intermit-
        tant, or constant?

3. Are symptoms related to movement?
    a. Body movement (in which direc-
        tions)?
    b. Head movement (in which direc-
        tions)?

4. Patient's general health
    a. Cardiovascular disorders?
    b. Metabolic disorders?
    c. Cervical neck disorders?
    d. Eyesight or eye movement?
    e. Any treatment with ototoxic drugs
        in the past?

5. Has patient ever lost consciousness?
    a. How long was patient unconscious?
    b. Was this related to or accompanied
        by dizziness?

6. Patient's hearing
    a. Have there been any changes or
        fluctuations in hearing?
        1) When?
        2) Which ear?
    b. Tinitus
        1) When?
        2) Which ear?

    c.   Feeling of fullness in the ears
        1)   When?
        2)   Which ear?
    d.   Is there a known perforation?

ENG Test Battery and the Audiologist's Role in Interpretation

The entire ENG test battery consists of the following:

> Tracking Tests--Pendular and OPK
>
> Positional Tests--in sitting and supine positions
>
> Hallpike Positioning Tests
>
> Bithermal Calorics

The test battery is done to provide information as to the probable location of the cause of vertigo. The test will in no way make a diagnosis; it will provide information to allow a diagnosis to be made, however. The ENG test battery must always be accompanied by a complete audiological test, including impedance testing, and by a thorough medical-otological examination. Combined with audiological-otological information, the ENG test battery is a powerful, localizing tool. Unfortunately, several unique situations exist with ENG that must be taken into consideration in the interpretation and reporting of test results.

The test is designed to determine if there is:

(a) any ocular-motor defect

(b) any spontaneous nystagmus

(c) any gaze nystagmus

(d) any positional nystagmus

(e)   any difference between vestibular
      system responses to calorics.

    In some clincial settings, measurements
may also be made to determine if a directional preponderance exists. The directional
preponderance test, however, is a weak test
and is not always included in ENG interpretation.

    Unfortunately   the   caloric   response
measurements do not differentiate between a
disorder within the vestibular end organ and
one affecting the vestibular portion of the
VIIIth nerve and/or the vestibular nucleus.
Therefore, the responses to calorics and any
asymmetry (a 20% difference between vestibular systems is considered a true asymmetry)
can be reported only in the following manner:

(1)   The calorics are normal and sym-
      metrical.

(2)   A unilateral weakness of a given
      amount exists showing a poorer left
      or right vestibular system.

(3)   A bilateral vestibular weakness
      exists.

    The   tracking   tests   and   findings   on
postional   tests   are   reported   as   follows:

(1)   OPK and Pendular tests are sym-
      metrical or asymmetrical, normal,
      or abnormal.

(2)   If a spontaneous nystagmus exists,
      its   degree   and   direction   is
      reported.

(3)   If a positional nystagmus exists,
      the position at which it occurs is

reported; any latency in response,
and whether or not the nystagmus
fatigues on repeat testing also are
reported.

The semantics of reporting ENG findings
are important. There is no difference in
vestibular function and thus ENG results
between a hypofunctioning vestibular system
secondary to Meniere's disease and a hypofunctioning system secondary to an acoustic
neuroma. The history, audiograms, and physician's physical findings, along with the ENG
test, lead to the final diagnosis. With this
in mind, the audiologist should carefully
word the ENG summary sheet. The summary of
findings should report all of these areas in
a clear and orderly manner.

The Appendix attached to this chapter
includes summary sheets that indicate the
manner in which various findings are reported
(Figs. 4-6). Note the manner in which indications for a pheripheral system disorder are
mentioned, as well as the wording used to
indicate disease even in the presence of a
normally responding vestibular system.

The attached Appendix also includes a
pretest instruction sheet, as well as some
essentials of history taking.

Summary

The audiologist is, in this author's
opinion, the logical individual to provide
accurate ENG testing and reporting of data.
This chapter has attempted to illustrate some
of the major considerations, that would not
have been found elsewhere in the literature,
of providing ENG in an audiological practice.
The selected bibliography will provide fur-

ther information relating to the specifics of
data interpretation. The information in this
chapter, along with adequate knowledge of the
ENG test battery, is meant to serve my colleagues well.

SUGGESTED READING

Barber H.: Positional nystagmus especially after head injury. Laryngoscope 74: 891, 1964

Barber H: Positional nystagmus: testing and interpretation. Trans Am Acad Opthalmol Otolaryngol 52:248-260, 1964

Barber HO, Stockwell CW: Manual of Electronystagmography. St. Louis, C. V. Mosby Company, 1976

Coats A: Directional preponderance and unilateral weakness. Ann Otol 74:655, 1965

Coats A: Directional preponderance and spontaneous nystagmus. Ann Otol Rhino Laryngal 75:1135, 1966

Coats AC: Manual of Electronystagmographic Technique. Houston, Texas, The Methodist Hospital, 1971, 67 pp

English GM: Otolaryngology, A Textbook. New York, Harper and Row, 1976, pp 77-113

Jongkees LBW: Vestibular tests. Arch Orolaryng 85:548, 1967

Jongkees LBW: Cervical vertigo. Laryngoscope 79:1473, 1969

Norris TM: Electronystagmography, in Northern J. (ed): Hearing Disorders. Little, Brown and Co., 1976, pp 53-65

Rubin W: Clinical electronystagmography. Laryngoscope 80:610-619, April 1970

Smith, C. R.: Measurement of nystagmus using electronystagmography (ENG). J Speech Hear Disord 32:2, May 1967

APPENDIX

CHAPTER IX

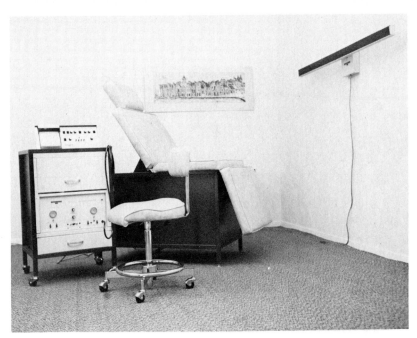

FIGURE 1

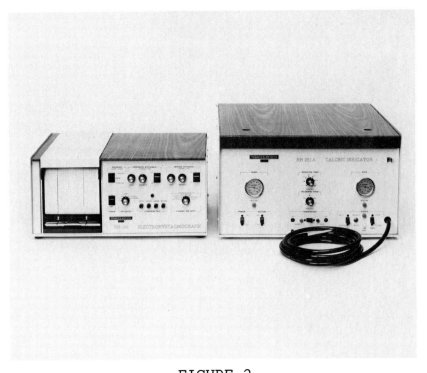

FIGURE 2

DARREL L. TETER, Ph.D. AND ASSOCIATES

Speech - Audiology
Language Disorders

191 East Orchard Road
Littleton, Colorado 80121
794-1133

6850 East Hampden Avenue
Denver, Colorado 80224
758-3415

BALANCE TEST INSTRUCTIONS

You are to be scheduled for a test of your balance mechanism. Certain medications often affect the result of these tests. In order to prevent this from happening, it will be necessary for you to NOT take any of the following medications or beverages for one day (24 Hours) before the time of your test appointment:

1. Sleeping Pills
2. Tranquilizers
3. Antihistamines
4. Barbiturates

5. Alcoholic Beverages
6. Anti-dizzy Pills
7. Sedatives
8. Muscle Relaxants

NO EATING 4 HOURS BEFORE THE TEST

NO COFFEE OR OTHER LIQUIDS 4 HOURS BEFORE THE TEST.

NO SMOKING 4 HOURS BEFORE THE TEST.

The balance test is a simple, painless procedure requiring about 2 hours. Electrodes will be taped near your eyes to make a tracing to determine if you have any balance problems related to head position or to your inner ear. Small amounts of both cool and warm water will be run into your oter ear canal. The cooling and warming effect of this water may make you a little dizzy. If it does, it will be over in a minute or two.

Please dress comfortably; women may desire to wear slacks.

FIGURE 3

DARREL L. TETER, Ph.D. AND ASSOCIATES

Speech - Audiology
Language Disorders

191 East Orchard Road
Littleton, Colorado 80121
794-1133

ENG SUMMARY

Date Tested: _____

6850 East Hampden Avenue
Denver, Colorado 80224
758-3415

TO: _____

Patients Name: _____

POSITIONAL TESTS: No Vertical nystagmus seen

SITTING: There is a right beating nystagmus in all head right positions. It shows latency and
fatigues.

LATERAL BODIES: There is a right beating nystagmus in body right position that shows latency
and fatigues.

SUPINE: There is a right beating nystagmus in head right positions that shows latency and
decay.

271

NECK TORSION: No nystagmus seen.

HALLPIKES: There is a right beating nystagmus in Hallpike head hanging right and in return to sitting from head hanging left (which would be a right head turn. It shows latency and fatigue.

PENDULAR TRACKING: Normal   OPTOKINETIC: Normal

COMMENTS ON POSITION TESTS: There is a right beating nystagmus in all head right positions which shows signs of latency and fatigue. We could not demonstrate this nystagmus to be related to a cervical neck disorder.

BITHERMAL CALORIC TESTS:

Stimulus	Post Irrigation		
	30 seconds	60 seconds	90 seconds
Right 44°	20°	18°	15°
Right 30°	15°	13°	10°
Left 44°	42°	30°	21°
Left 30°	25°	24°	18°

FIGURE 4

(ENG Summary continued)

PATIENT'S SUBJECTIVE IMPRESSION OF CALORICS: Calorics reproduced clinical symptoms.

WAS PATIENT ABLE TO INHIBIT INDUCED NYSTAGMUS? Yes   WHEN? R 44°C and L 44°

UNILATERAL WEAKNESS

Right 44°	53	
Right 30°	38	36%
	91	
Left 44°	93	
Left 30°	67	64%
	160	
TOTAL =	251	
DIFFERENCE	28	

DIRECTIONAL PREPONDERANCE

Right 44°	53	
Left 30°	67	48%
	120	
Left 44°	93	
Right 30°	38	52%
	131	
TOTAL =	251	
DIFFERENCE	4	

SUMMARY: Bithermal calorics reveal a 28% difference with the right vestibular system giving a weaker response. This coupled with the positional findings are indicative of a right vestibular system disorder.

273

DARREL L. TETER, Ph.D. AND ASSOCIATES

Speech - Audiology
Language Disorders

191 East Orchard Road
Littleton, Colorado 80121
794-1133

6850 East Hampden Avenue
Denver, Colorado 80224
758-3415

ENG SUMMARY

Date Tested: _____

TO: _____

Patients Name: _____

POSITIONAL TESTS: No Vertical nystagmus seen

SITTING: There is a spontaneous right beating nystagmus of approximately 7° that is unaltered
by changes in head positions.

SUPINE: Spontaneous right beating nystagmus of approximately 7° that is unaltered by changes
in head position.

275

HALLPIKES: Spontaneous right beating nystagmus of approximately 7° that is unaltered by changes in head position.

PENDULAR TRACKING: Abnormal   OPTOKINETIC: Abnormal

COMMENTS ON POSITION TESTS: There is a spontaneous right beating nystagmus of approximately 7° in all positions.

BITHERMAL CALORIC TESTS:

Stimulus		Post Irrigation	
	30 seconds	60 seconds	90 seconds
Right 44°	27°	25°	22°
Right 30°	8°	6°	3°
Left 44°	13°	11°	8°
Left 30°	22°	20°	17°

FIGURE 5

(ENG Summary continued)

PATIENT'S SUBJECTIVE IMPRESSION OF CALORICS: Calorics reproduced clinical symptoms.

WAS PATIENT ABLE TO INHIBIT INDUCED NYSTAGMUS? Yes   WHEN?   R 44°C and L 44°

UNILATERAL WEAKNESS

Right 44°	74	
Right 30°	17	50%
	91	
Left 44°	32	
Left 30°	59	50%
	91	
TOTAL =	182	
DIFFERENCE	0	

DIRECTIONAL PREPONDERANCE

Right 44°	_____
Left 30°	_____
Left 44°	_____
Right 30°	_____
TOTAL =	_____
DIFFERENCE	_____

SUMMARY: Bithermal calorics are strong and symmetrical. We see no evidence of a vestibular system disorder, however, there is a spontaneous nystagmust present; a Central Nervous System disorder must be ruled out.

DARREL L. TETER, Ph.D. AND ASSOCIATES

Speech - Audiology
Language Disorders

6850 East Hampden Avenue
Denver, Colorado 80224
758-3415

191 East Orchard Road
Littleton, Colorado 80121
794-1133

ENG SUMMARY

TO: _____   Patients Name: _____   Date Tested: _____

POSITIONAL TESTS: No Vertical nystagmus seen

SITTING: No vertical nystagmus seen. No spontaneous or positional nystagmus seen.

SUPINE: No nystagmus seen.

279

HALLPIKES: No nystagmus seen.

PENDULAR TRACKING: Normal   OPTOKINETIC: Normal

COMMENTS ON POSITION TESTS: No nystagmus seen in any position.

BITHERMAL CALORIC TESTS:

Stimulus

	30 seconds	Post Irrigation 60 seconds	90 seconds
Right 44°	22°	16°	15°
Right 30°	15°	13°	10°
Left 44°	21°	18°	10°
Left 30°	12°	13°	8°

FIGURE 6

(ENG Summary continued)

PATIENT'S SUBJECTIVE IMPRESSION OF CALORICS: Calorics did not reproduce clincial symptons.

WAS PATIENT ABLE TO INHIBIT INDUCED NYSTAGMUS?   Yes   WHEN?   R 44°C and L 44°

UNILATERAL WEAKNESS

Right 44°   53
Right 30°   38   53%
             ——
             91

Left 44°   49
Left 30°   33   47%
             ——
             82

TOTAL =   173
DIFFERENCE   6

DIRECTIONAL PREPONDERANCE

Right 44°   53
Left 30°   33   50%
             ——
             86

Left 44°   49
Right 30°   38   50%
             ——
             87

TOTAL =   173
DIFFERENCE   0

SUMMARY: Bithermal calorics are strong and symmetrical. We see no evidence of a vestibular system disorder at this time.

CHAPTER X

DISPENSING HEARING AIDS IN
PRIVATE PRACTICE

Vernon C. Bragg, Ph.D.

Discussion of the role of the audiologist in hearing aid dispensing has been lengthy, loud, and often bitter. It has also been carried out primarily between non-audiologist dispensers and non-dispensing audiologists. Very little has been said by the so-called "dispensing audiologists," perhaps because they are so few in number and perhaps because of the attitudes regarding dispensing which are held by some of their colleagues within the profession. Any audiologist who enters or considers entering private practice must give some thought to whether or not he will dispense hearing aids, and, if he does, the method and mechanics of the procedure.

It is the purpose of this chapter to present some ideas and procedures that have been developed during almost 30 years in the field of audiology, the last four and a half of which have been spent as a private-practice dispensing audiologist. Because these are only my own personal opinions and are based on my perceptions of personal experiences, I shall depart from the usual practice of providing references, tables, and illustrations for others' works. The experiences were my own and the conclusions are my own. Although most of what I have learned in these many years has been taught by others, only I may be held responsible for the conclusions which I have reached.

Should the Audiologist Enter
Private Practice?

First, one must consider whether the
audiologist should have a private practice at
all, or whether he should work for a salary
in a university, community clinic, or physician's office as do the great majority of his
colleagues. The choice, of course, is an
individual one, and many may not have the
choice of private practice for a variety of
reasons, not least of which may be financial.
It is the author's opinion that if audiology
is to survive and prosper as a profession,
our major thrust must be toward training
audiologists who will be capable of private
practice, and doing everything possible to
make private practice one of their practical
options.

A profession whose practitioners are
unable to stand alone and independent must
sooner or later lose its standing as a profession and be reduced to technician level.
In such a position, the audiologist may
develop very high-level information regarding
the patient's condition and needs, but the
final interpretation of this information and
the application of remedial action lies with
others; namely, the person or organization
that pays the audiologist's salary, the
physician who carries out the treatment or
performs the surgery, or the person who
provides and services the recommended hearing
aid. For his work, the audiologist may be
paid an appropriate salary and enjoy the
serenity and security of a job, but he is not
in the same position as the private practitioner because his relationship with the
patient is dependent upon some third person
or board which may alter or discontinue that
relationship at its pleasure. Only in private practice may we truly say that one is "my
patient," and only in this situation is the

relationship dependent only upon the patient and the practioner.

Should the Audiologist Dispense Hearing Aids?

In considering private practice, one must also judge the ethical factors involved in hearing aid dispensing if he plans to offer these services. For answers, he must search his own beliefs and test his own strengths. Above and beyond those restrictions placed on him by the American Speech and Hearing Association rules of ethical conduct are one's own moral convictions.

Regardless of whether a hearing aid is sold for a "fee" or a "profit," the fact is that the audiologist will receive money for fitting and dispensing that aid which he would not receive if he did not carry out these functions. If this consideration is likely to play an important part in the audiologist's decision to recommend an aid or not to recommend an aid, then he MUST NOT dispense hearing aids. These same considerations, of course, face the surgeon, the attorney, and all other professionals. The person who would perform unneeded surgery for a fee or recommend a lawsuit to his client because he will be paid for handling that suit, or who believes that he may be overly tempted to do these things, should avoid these professions for his own and the profession's good. No other rule of ethics is as important as this, and this takes precedence over all. Other rules of ethics may have a great effect on you and your practice for better or for worse, but you must assure yourself that you are able to give your patient the best of which you are capable without allowing financial considerations to affect your decisions unduly. If you can do

this, you will have no professional problems
in this area. As for ASHA's rules for dispensing, they often seem to be childish
attempts by which we try to assure ourselves
of our own honesty, but they are relatively
simple to abide by if we have faith in our
own individual trustworthiness. Their omis-
sion of general rules of referral procedures
is more regrettable and potentially more
stifling of private practice (and therefore
of audiology as a profession) than any restrictions which apply. More of this later.

Finally, the decision as to whether
audiologists should dispense hearing aids
depends upon the alternatives. One may well
answer this question by asking another: "Who
better?" No other professional has spent as
much time and effort in the study of hearing
as a phenomenon which may undergo a variety
of deviations from normal, the many manifes-
tations which these changes may bring about,
their effects upon the expression and reception of speech and language, and the nonmedi-
cal methods of reducing or eliminating the
possible handicapping results of non-normal
hearing function. Included in these studies
are many concerned with amplification and its
effects upon normal and abnormal hearing.

Arguments by hearing aid dealer organizations and certain individual dealers
imply that the audiologist is not qualified
to fit hearing aids and should be forbidden
by law from dispensing. Such arguments must
be based upon the contention that six years'
(minimum) professional study should disqual-
ify the person from applying that which he
has studied, or that audiological training
makes one less qualified than the person who
has no such training. This specious contention is debunked by those same organizations
when they set up membership requirements
based upon basic audiological information,

hire audiologists to teach courses to their applicants, attend audiological seminars, and use the title "Hearing Aid Audiologist."

The above is not to say that the non-audiologist hearing aid dispenser is always in the wrong in his disagreements with the audiologist, nor is he necessarily lacking in the formal and informal training necessary for his job. Many such dealers have accumulated many hours of college-level audiological training to supplement their practical experience, which is often considerable. At the same time, many of our university programs in Audiology appear to be woefully lacking in information and expertise about hearing aids. One is often shocked at our shortcomings and apparent lack of interest in this most important area of our responsibility. Certainly, a master's or doctor's degree in audiology may not be relied upon to make one a proficient fitter of hearing aids. It is, however, an excellent starting place.

If an audiologist is to accept the awesome responsibility of counseling hard-of-hearing patients toward maximum rehabilitation, honesty to himself and to his patient demands that he gain all possible knowledge about these instruments, their fitting, and their effects on the patient and his hearing. This applies whether he intends to dispense hearing aids or not. Auditory rehabilitation is the ultimate responsibility of the audiologist, and the hearing aid is a most important part of the rehabilitation process in a great majority of cases. It is often the only help available to the patient with sensorineural hearing loss. The audiologist who does not take every opportunity to advance his knowledge in this area, or who relinquishes his responsibilities to others who may not be well trained and who are not bound by the same rules of ethical practice,

might well refrain from private practice.
The patient who pays for audiological counseling rightfully demands that the audiologist be prepared with answers to his questions about all aspects of the rehabilitation
program.

Having decided that he is prepared to
enter private practice, the audiologist must
next determine if such a venture is possible
and practical for him. The answer to this
question may well depend upon his answer
regarding hearing aid dispensing. In a great
many situations, it may be impossible to
develop a private practice without dispensing
hearing aids. Much of the practice and much
of the financing may depend upon hearing aid
evaluation and fitting. It appears to the
author that there are few solvent private
practices in audiology that do not include
hearing aid fitting as a part of their income-
producing activities. It is difficult to
imagine any but the most exceptional situation in which "diagnostic evaluations" alone
would support a practice. A large enough
clientele in speechreading and auditory
training may provide sufficient work for the
private practitioner, but hearing aid fitting
remains a vital part of the rehabilitation in
most cases, and should best be accomplished
by an audiologist capable of accurate measurement and dispensing. He, of course,
should be properly compensated for his time
and expertise.

Can It Be Done?

Once we have established that the audiologist should have the option of dispensing
hearing aids in his practice, the question
arises as to its feasibility, or, "Can it be
done?" The answer to this most important
question cannot be an unqualified "Yes," but

neither should it be considered an impossible task. It is probably true that more young audiologists have failed in attempts at dispensing hearing aids than have succeeded. Private practice is not the rule within our profession, and many factors contribute to success or failure. More than one professor of audiology has told me, "Audiology is not a self-supporting profession. It cannot pay for itself, and must be supported by an organization, agency, or a medical practice." Perhaps this is one of the important reasons why we have not progressed in the area of private practice as we should. Our teachers are not experienced in private practice and often consider it impossible. Our programs do not prepare us for private practice, and seldom even mention the multitude of problems presented by the business aspects of any private professional venture. Finally, most of us do not enter audiology with any thought of financial gain. Anyone so naive as to study in this field for the purpose of "making money" must surely be too stupid to pass entrance examinations for the universities where it is taught. Most of us, therefore, are woefully unprepared to take on the direction of an operation which involves both a profession and a business. Few, too, are financially able to hire a business expert to take over these duties. Still, the details of purchasing, bill paying, accounting, planning, public relations, and collections, and all the myriad activities of a business, must be handled if the doors are to be kept open and the professional activities allowed to grow.

The difficulties faced by the young private practice aspirant are enormous, especially since he is breaking almost new ground. Unlike the new physician or attorney, he has no established and proven pattern to follow. The doctor or lawyer knows that

his practice can be successful, and he knows
what must be done, at least in a general way.
It is also true that lending institutions
know the success rate of these professions,
and banks are willing and anxious to lend
support to well-qualified practitioners.

The following pages will discuss some of
the problems we face in setting up a private
practice which includes hearing aid dispensing. Throughout this discussion, the reader
should keep in mind that such a practice is
possible to accomplish, and that it offers
the audiologist a most rewarding situation in
which he can apply the best of his knowledge
in working with patients who need and want
his services and show their trust in him by
continuing the patient-practitioner relationship. Other professions have met the challenge of standing alone in private practice.
We stand today in a situation very similar to
that which faced psychology not too many
years ago. Now, independent private practice
is a commonly accepted and viable option in
psychology. It must become so for audiology
if we are to attain the stature to which we
have so long aspired.

Problems in Private Practice Dispensing

Visibility. Perhaps our greatest difficulty as audiologists entering private practice is that of letting the public know what
we do and what we offer. Every citizen knows
what a doctor, a lawyer, or a dentist is, and
what he does. He also knows where to find
one when he needs one. Very few even know
what an audiologist is or what unique talents
he has and what services he provides. When
the potential patient realizes that he may
have a problem with hearing, he sometimes
(though not always) goes to his physician for

treatment or advice. Often if his doctor
refers him to an audiologist, the patient
cannot understand why he should have to pay
someone else to tell him he has a hearing
loss when that is why he went to his doctor
in the first place. If the audiologist then
tells him that he needs amplification, but
must go to yet a third person for the help he
needs, he may logically give up the whole
idea or conclude that somewhere along the
line, something is missing. In many cases,
of course, the doctor will not refer him to
an audiologist at all. He may simply tell
him that he has a "nerve type" loss which
cannot be helped. Or, he may tell him to see
if he can find a hearing aid which will help.

If the person decides, as far too many
of them do, that he will by-pass medical
advice, he is most likely to turn to the
commercial hearing aid dealer. Assuming that
he knows what an audiologist is, and has hope
of help from that sector, how is he to find
the private practitioner? If he looks in the
advertisements, he will find the hearing aid
dealer. If he asks a friend, he most likely
will be given the brand name of a hearing
aid. The efforts of ASHA and state Speech
and Hearing Associations to obtain recogni-
tion for audiologists have been directed
almost exclusively in behalf of community and
university speech and hearing clinics. I am
unable to recall any such advertisement or
public announcement which mentions the private practitioner; I certainly have seen none
that indicate that audiologists dispense
hearing aids. This despite the fact that
many dispensing audiologists save the hearing
aid purchaser hundreds of dollars and provide
professional guidance based on intimate
experience with hearing aids and their use of
a kind which is not available to any others
in the field. In other professions, the
private practitioner is not left so alone by

his organization. The American Dental Association urges the public through massive advertising to "see your dentist," and the ADA approves (or presumably disapproves) all things to do with tooth care--pastes, brushes, etc. The American Medical Association makes policy and headlines simultaneously by public statements regarding the practice of medicine and the usefulness of certain drugs, procedures, and appliances as they affect our health. Even the National Hearing Aid Society enlists the help of hard-of-hearing celebrities to publicize successful hearing aid help provided by their members.

Referral policies. It is most regrettable from the private practice audiologist's standpoint that ASHA and state organizations have no referral policies to provide guidelines for their members. In all other professions, referrals are made, as far as is possible, within the profession. Thus, the internist refers his patient needing surgery to another physician who specializes in surgery. The corporation lawyer whose client asks for information on income taxes refers the client to another attorney and not to H. and R. Block or the Sears Income Tax desk. In this way, the professional reflects a knowledge of the worth of his own profession and an interest in the welfare of his client. He assures himself that his client will receive professional treatment from a fellow professional who meets the same standards of training, experience, and ethics which he himself must meet. It is a part of the professional's responsibility to his client to refer to the best available source for services which he himself does not provide, and he can expect such referrals from others within his profession. Indeed, most physicians would have found private practice impossible to enter had they not been able to depend upon referrals from collegues at least during the tough early months of practice.

As far as I know, there has been no rule expressed by an speech and hearing organization regarding referral practices for audiologists and speech/language pathologists. Nothing in ASHA's regulations mentions the desirability of referring patients needing speech pathology to a qualified member of the organization, or one needing hearing aid counseling to an audiologist. Many of our colleagues are taught that a direct referral for a hearing aid is somehow unethical. In some clinics, the audiologist may go only so far as to give the patient a list of persons who sell hearing aids. Many of these lists do not even mention the dispensing audiologist's degree or qualifications, nor is the patient told that, because much of the work has already been done, he may save a great deal of money by going to the audiologist for his aid. Although most audiologists try to give their patients this vital information, even if it means stretching clinic rules a bit, others apparently consider the private dispensing audiologist as threatening competition or as slightly "shady" for dispensing hearing aids. These may well be the same audiologists who have for many years been crying out the need for less expensive hearing aids, better qualified dispensers, and stronger ethical practices regulations for the dispenser. It is my opinion that a consistent policy of referral by audiologists and speech pathologists to others within their own ranks would result in a great many more openings within these fields, better handling of our patients, and a marvelous reduction in the cost of hearing aids.

Competition. In private practice, as in any other venture, competition should be

considered as an impetus to better service
and not a difficulty to be faced. However,
the recent bitterness between certain audiologists and some of the hearing aid dealers
has led to unfortunate expressions of competition which may affect the audiologist who
wants to enter the hearing aid field. One
may expect his referral sources to be told
how audiology intends to take over the practice of medicine or of how the dispensing
audiologist adds "hidden charges" to his
bills, charging outrageous fees for services
which the dealer gives free. They may be
told, at the same time, that he cannot stay
in practice at the low prices he charges, so
he must soon have to go out of business,
leaving his patient with no source of service
for his hearing aid. Patients will be
visited and told these same stories, which
are largely the "party line" of dealer organizations rather than the personal convictions of the individual dealer. Letters may
be written to state licensing boards and to
ASHA outlining supposed breaches of ethics by
the audiologist. Fortunately, such tactics
are not too common and are ineffective enough
that they soon fade away. It may be expected
that as more and more audiologists begin
dispensing hearing aids and the public learns
more about these activities, less and less
bitterness will exist between audiologist and
non-audiologist dispensers.

Competition of another sort is often
experienced by the private practitioner,
although this is often very constructive
competition. Many university programs and
physicians' offices are dependent upon the
same source for patients as is the private
audiologist. Although it may seem very
difficult to compete with a clinic which is
supported by tax money, or with an audiological practice financed by a medical practice,
these should pose no great problem in a well-

planned practice. It is obviously unwise to attempt private practice in a small town where the university clinic and/or the local otologist provides all the needed services in audiology. If there is no need for the services, competition will not matter one way or the other. If the services are needed and are provided better and/or more reasonably, then such competition will be both invigorating and supportive.

Financing. This is always a problem, and is often the cause for failure in audiology as well as in other fields of endeavor. The basic cost of equipping and furnishing even a small office space can represent a substantial outlay. Audiometers, sound rooms, impedance meters, typewriters, desks, hearing aid test equipment and stock, repair facilities, and dozens of other expensive items are needed to begin operations. Overhead in the form of telephone, rent, help, etc. must also be paid from the beginning. Of course, living expenses continue to go on whether one's income is sufficient or not. Unless proper financing is available, one should seek other avenues than simply opening an office. If you do not have sufficient funds, check on your ability to borrow before committing what you do have.

FDA Hearing Aid Regulations. These regulations, which became effective on August 25, 1977, impose strict controls on the manufacturer of hearing aids. These have had an effect on hearing aid prices, and may have an even greater effect in the future. Because of the added tests required on each hearing aid, the stringent performance limits which an aid must meet if it is to be sold, and the additional information which must be provided to the consumer, most hearing aid manufacturers have raised the wholesale price of their products. Regulations affecting the

dispenser should be no problem for the audiologist dispenser, since they call for no
unreasonable actions. Briefly, the new
regulations require medical (preferably
otological) clearance before a hearing aid
can be sold, rented, or loaned. Because
audiologists have always held to the view
that such medical clearance is desirable and
this has long been ASHA policy, I see no
conflict or problem. The patient must be
told of the advisibility of physician clearance, but he may waive the examination except
in the presence of one or more of several
conditions which would require otological
referral in any case. Persons under the age
of 18 may not waive medical examination under
any circumstances.

Some Recommendations

Although I consider my own private
practice to be successful, I lay no claim to
knowing "How to Set Up a Successful Practice
in Dispensing Audiology" by any means. My
own success, such as it is, depends upon a
great number of fortuitous circumstances. I
practice in the tenth largest city in the
nation, where I have lived for over six years
and have known all of the other audiologists
and most of the otologists personally. I
receive strong help from all of these and
others, and third-party programs helped
greatly in the beginning, as they continue to
do. I was guided to a good selection of
office space by a friend with a great deal of
experience in the hearing aid field; office
overhead is low enough to allow me to charge
much less than most offices do while still
maintaining the quality which I deem necessary. Initial financing did not pose a
problem.

In spite of the fact that I have no success formula to offer, and that I know little of business procedures, there are certain principles and observations which I would like to pass on to the audiologist who may be considering a practice which includes hearing aid dispensing. I shall discuss these as they come to mind in hopes that they may prove helpful as general guides.

1. First, decide if you really want to dispense hearing aids. The job involves much more than the hearing aid evaluation. It takes dedicated patience in working with people who may understand very little of the technical information they need to know to use the aid. It takes a great deal of time spent in such things as checking batteries and making earmolds and changing tubes and explaining, explaining, explaining. Broken aids must be repaired or sent in for repair. Records must be kept and bills must be paid. For every hearing aid dispensed, you may expect four or five visits for rechecking, adjusting, and more explaining. And you will find that many hearing aid purchasers expect much more from a hearing aid than they should reasonably expect. The advertising has told them to expect it.

2. Study hearing aids. If your only experience has been in hearing aid evaluations at your college clinic, there are many things you probably could profit from learning. Can you read the specification sheets and translate them into the information needed to help the patient? Do you know what effect you may

expect from earmold modifications? Do you know the advantages and disadvantages of the various types of aids--behind the ear, in the ear, CROS, etc.? Learn to cut and stretch tubing, and to make earmolds. Hearing aids will now become important tools of your trade, and you must know as much about them as you can.

3.   Contact manufacturers. The makers of hearing aids can be most helpful in all aspects of your practice as they apply to hearing aids. Their representatives are extremely knowledgeable about their own aids and those of their competitors. Many of these men have spent years learning about aids and visiting clinics and dealers all over the country. From them you can learn about fitting and adjusting as well as all the many small but important "tricks" for making a fitting more acceptable or for handling the business end of your practice. These men are invaluable to the dispenser, and often possess a world of knowledge which we need. It is better to select a few hearing aids to work with from those you judge to be best and those represented by men with whom you can work well than to try to fit all brands. One soon learns to feel easy with a certain number of aids, preferring perhaps an eyeglass aid from one line and an in-the-ear aid from another. Most companies no longer demand "exclusive" representation, and their representatives will help with all your problems.

4. Selecting office space. Because most of your business will come from referrals, it is imperative that the office be easily available. This usually means that an office in a large medical center is best. It is surprisingly difficult to assure that a patient will accept a referral, especially if it involves extra effort. A patient may come to your office if it is in the same building or very near that of the referring physician or audiologist, but may refuse to go across town. Proximity to referral sources is extremely important.

5. Building referral sources. Direct contact is the best way to develop referrals. Before opening, of course, an announcement should be sent to all possible referral sources--otologists, audiologists, speech and hearing centers, pediatricians, and other professionals. Those mentioned should be visited, if possible, and apprised of the services you intend to offer. Ask for referrals frankly and assure them that you will do your best to provide the best possible service to their patients. Some physicians and audiologists are anxious to know that they will receive a report and that the patient will return to them for further counseling and treatment. Reports should be brief and appropriate.

    While the life blood of a practice is professional referral, especially for the first year or until patient referral builds, misunderstandings are possible.

Because you do not receive any or many patients on referral from a certain clinic or professional, do not assume that you are being ignored. As mentioned before, the patient makes the decision, and simply because you have been recommended does not mean that he is obligated to visit you. Also, do not expect to get all the referrals from all professional sources, even if you feel your services are the best available. Doctors may be reluctant to stop referring to a dealer who has been providing satisfactory service to his patients for some time and who shows faith in that doctor by sending his own clients to him when they require medical treatment. Referrals will certainly come to the practitioner who can provide the best possible service, and who honestly gives his best to all patients. Never refuse an opportunity to address local professional and club meetings about your practice, and always offer as much help as you can to the individual or the organization who is concerned with hearing problems. The strongest referral source is people who know your capabilities and your willingness to help.

A final word about referrals. Too many private practices have been built on the promise and expectation of referrals which fail to develop, and these practices fail because of this. Because you have polled the possible referral sources and received enthusiastic estimates from each as to how many

patients he will send you, do not
build all your hopes on this
source. For one or more reasons,
those patients may not reach your
office, at least for a very long
time after being "sent."

6. Alternative ways to establish a
    practice. It is not always neces-
    sary (or possible) to finance the
    development of your own practice,
    even by going deep into debt.
    Other methods for getting started
    have been successful at times. It
    may be possible to buy a share in
    an existing practice which is ready
    to expand, or to work in another's
    practice with an arrangement that
    will lead to partnership after a
    certain length of time, or when a
    certain level of increase has been
    shown. A few audiologists have
    been employed by otologists with
    the option to buy the audiological
    portion of the practice over a
    period of time. While these prac-
    tices are usually tied to the
    otological practice, and are there-
    fore not private practices in the
    strictest sense of the word, they
    offer a great deal more freedom of
    action and opportunity to develop
    than do straight salaried arrange-
    ments which may be terminated at
    will, and where salary is dependent
    upon agreement rather than upon
    earned income.

    In any arrangement involving
    more than one professional, whether
    it be partnership or employee/
    employer, one must expect his share
    to be dependent upon that portion
    of the practice which he himself

"generates." Private practice in any form must be self-supporting, since it does not depend upon taxes or donations for operating expenses and profit. Therefore, it is not reasonable to expect full partnership and an equal share of the practice unless and until your own efforts attract an equal share of the patients and the revenue. The same applies to a salaried position within another's practice. Unless your presence in the practice accounts for at least enough patient activity to "carry your load," your services are an added expense rather than an advantage. Secretarial help, nursing, and receptionist activities are services which may be required and which do not necessarily attract patients. The professional in private practice, whether his own or someone else's, must attract patients in sufficient numbers to support his own work and all the supplementary services and accoutrements attendant on their presentation. This is the challenge of private enterprise, and this is the mark which one must be ready to meet. The audiologist who is able and willing to offer enough of himself to justify his patients' continued support will gain more from meeting the challenge than he can have expected. It is this author's belief that the audiologist who can provide the patient with professional guidance through the trials of rehabilitation from hearing loss offers a service deserving of independent private practice.

A vital part of that rehabilitation process is the fitting and dispensing of a proper hearing aid, and the counseling, teaching, checking, and explaining its use and limitations. The audiologist is prepared through formal training to learn the necessary skills to accomplish this task better than the members of any other profession. If he cannot, with his background of knowledge, improve upon the art of hearing aid fitting, then he might well leave private practice to others. The audiologist who undertakes the dispensing of hearing aids carries with him the responsibility to do more than simply to carry on the present state of the art. His knowledge must be applied to the improvement of the hearing aid user's lot and to the development of additional information which will lead to better hearing aids and better fitting procedures than those which are now available.

Index

Accounting, 35
Adequate financial return, 13
Administrator, 34, 42, 187
Advertising, 212
Agency, 53, 54, 57–62, 138, 295
Allen, J. M., 133
American Academy of Private Practice in
    Speech Pathology and Audiology,
    1–3, 74, 195
American Speech and Hearing
    Association, 1, 2, 4, 10, 14, 23, 73,
    77, 224, 286, 291, 292, 293, 296
Announcements, 14–17, 212
Aphasia, 12, 96, 159, 161, 162
Aram, D. M., 116, 121, 130, 134
Articulation, 95
Audiology
    clinical aspects, 191
    student, 196
Audiological testing, 91, 197, 200, 201,
    213, 215, 216, 217, 222, 228, 234,
    235

Bad debts, 29, 30, 32
Bangs, T., 133
Barber, H., 263
Battin, R. R., 1, 5
Beginning practice, 10
Billing, 27, 28, 202, 225
Bluemel, C. S., 1
Brain, R., 174
Brodnitz, 1
Budget, 155, 199, 204
Butler, K., 115, 133

Calibration, 223, 224
California Speech Pathologists and
    Audiologists in Private Practice, 3
Cambell, C. P., 87
Capital, 9
Carlin, M., 85, 87

Certificate of Clinical Competence, 4, 77,
    147, 195, 196
Clinician, 4, 11
Clinical areas, 3
Clinical Fellowship Year, 195
Clinical management, 3
Clinical skills, 1, 4, 9
Coats, A. C., 263
Collections, 29, 289
Competence, 3
Consultant, 10, 13
Contracts, 13, 73, 148, 149, 150, 151,
    152, 172, 182
Corporation, 11, 48, 49
Cowdry, E. V., 137, 138, 141, 145, 150,
    174, 175

Darley, F. L., 133
D'Asaro, M. L., 4, 5
Deaf education, 216
Director
    medical, 19, 185
    other, 154, 155
Disorders, 3

Eisenson, J., 160
Electronystagmography, 224, 241
    equipment, 241, 242, 246, 247, 249,
        250, 251, 252, 253, 254, 255, 261
    testing, 241, 242, 243, 244, 245, 247,
        255, 256, 257, 258, 259, 260, 268,
        271, 273, 275, 276, 277, 279, 281
Emerick, 121, 133
English, G. M., 263
English, R. E., 116, 133
Equipment
    clinical, 23, 24, 198, 200, 206, 207,
        208, 218, 219, 223, 224
    office, 21, 24, 199, 209, 210
Espir, M., 160
Ethics, 4, 14, 73, 83, 196, 220, 285

305

Expert witness, 74, 76, 78, 79, 82, 85, 86, 201

Facility, 19
Fees, 10, 30, 31, 32, 33, 34, 199, 200, 201, 228, 229, 247, 285
Financing, 295
Fox, D. R., 116, 133
Froeschels, E., 1
Fuller, C., 134

Gay, R. M., 135
Geriatric groups, 13
Glueck, S., 87
Good, R., 133
Goodglass, H., 160
Growth potential, 13, 42, 43

Hammond, K. R., 133
Hatten, J. T., 121, 133
Health care services, 2
Hearing aid, 213, 221, 284, 297, 298
Hearing aid dealer, 286
Hearing aid dispensing, 283, 285, 286, 287, 288, 289, 290, 294, 296, 297, 303
Hearing aid evaluation, 214, 229
Hearing aid regulations, 295
Hearing conservation, 198
Hearing screening program, 198
Helping professions, 2
Holidays, 199
Home health
   evaluation, 165–167
   history, 137–138
   organizations, 142–143
   personnel, 148
Huber, J. T., 116, 127, 133

Insurance carrier, 57, 61, 122, 123, 125, 202, 203, 238
   government, 124, 202
   liability, 186, 248, 249
Investment, 9, 44–47, 246
Itemizing, 202, 238

Jerger, J., 116, 133
Johnson, W., 116, 121, 133

Jones, W. P., 126, 134
Jong Kees, L. B., 263

Kellner, 87
Klopfler, 116, 127, 134
Knepflar, 115, 116, 119, 124, 127, 130, 133
Knight, P. D., 1, 2, 5

Landis, B. A., 1, 5
Language disorders, 12, 97
Laquaite, J., 134
Legislation
   national, 2, 53, 54
Lewin, M. H., 29, 51
Liebson, H. A., 74, 77, 87
Lillywhite, H. S., 116, 133
Living expenses, 9
Location, 22

Mayman, M., 134
Medicare, 54, 55, 56, 57, 122, 125, 139, 202, 233, 238
Meetings, 41, 199
Merrill, P. W., 134
Moore, M. V., 116, 134
Morris, W., 129, 134

Nation, J. E., 116, 120, 130, 134
Norris, J. M., 263

Osgood, C., 160
Otology, 216, 229
Overhead, 34, 36, 226
Overholser, W., 87

Pannbacker, M., 116, 134
Parent, 4
Partnership, 10, 44, 301
Part time practice, 10
Patient, 4, 10, 11, 18
Peer review, 169
Penfield, W., 160
Personnel, 20, 36–39, 45, 210
Porch, B., 87
Practice
   group, 10, 18, 19

independent, 1, 3, 19, 42, 191, 197, 215
individual, 11, 13
private, 1, 2, 4, 9, 10, 14, 283, 284
solo, 10, 19, 44, 290, 302
Practitioner, 1–4, 10–14, 18, 117, 283, 284
Privileged communication, 84
Professional meetings, 40, 41
Progress reports, 61, 124
Proprietorship, 11
Provider number, 59

Quadfasel, F., 160

Rada, R. T., 87
Records
  clinical, 171
  financial, 28
  medical, 170
Referral source, 14, 40, 156, 158, 211, 299, 300
Reports
  basic, considering, 117, 125
  diagnostic, 120, 130, 178
  specialized, 120, 122
Retirement, 44, 46, 47
Rister, A., 133
Riviere, M., 134
Roberts, L., 160
Rubin, W., 263
Russel, W., 160

Salaries, 34, 43, 227, 284, 301
Sanders, H. J., 121, 135
Schedule, 33, 93
School age children, 13
Shaw, H., 129, 135
Sick leave, 33, 199

Sisson, R. F., 129, 135
Skillen, M. E., 129, 135
Smith, C. R., 263
Social Security, 53, 55
Space, 20, 22, 204, 205, 225, 247, 299
Specialization, 9
Speech and hearing services, 4
Speech and language testing, 92, 94, 97
Speech pathology care plan, 180
Speech pathologists and audiologists in private practice, 2, 3
Spriestersbach, D., 133
State Department of Public Health, 55, 61
Steinberg, F. U., 137, 138, 141, 145, 150, 175
Structural defects, 12, 95
Strunk, W., 126, 135
Stuttering, 1, 2, 94, 95
Summers, R., 1, 5

Tallent, N., 116, 126, 127, 135
Telephone answering service, 21
Therapeutic relationship, 4
Transference, 4
Travis, L. E., 159, 160, 163, 175
Teuber, H., 170, 175

Utilization review, 168, 185, 186

Vacation, 40, 199
Van Riper, C., 1, 5
Voice, 96

Webster, A. M., 4
Weis, D., 1
Wepman, J. N., 74, 77, 87
White, E. B., 135
Woodford, F. P., 135

a
b
c
d
e
8 f
9 g
0 h
1 i
8 2 j